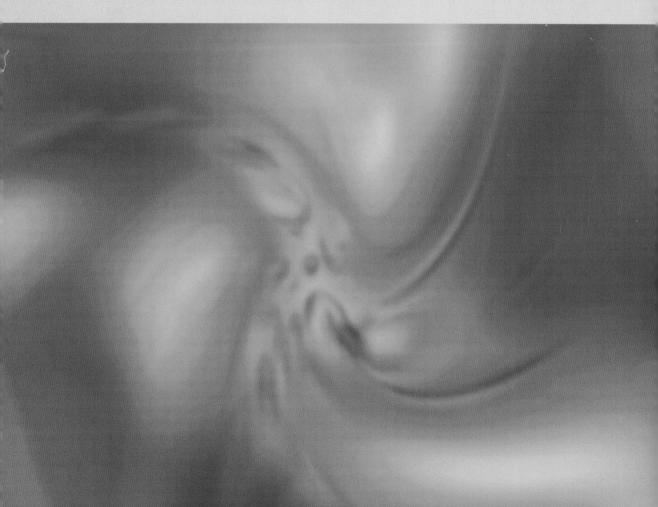

✓ GALLUP
MAJOR TRENDS & EVENTS
The Pulse of Our Nation: 1900 to the Present

Health Care

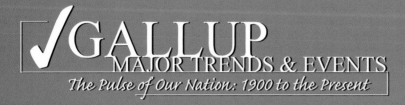

GALLUP
MAJOR TRENDS & EVENTS
The Pulse of Our Nation: 1900 to the Present

Abortion

Drug & Alcohol Abuse

Health Care

Immigration

Marriage & Family Issues

Obesity

Race Relations

Technology

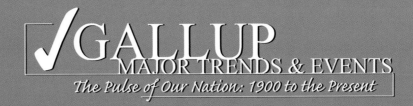

GALLUP
MAJOR TRENDS & EVENTS
The Pulse of Our Nation: 1900 to the Present

Health Care

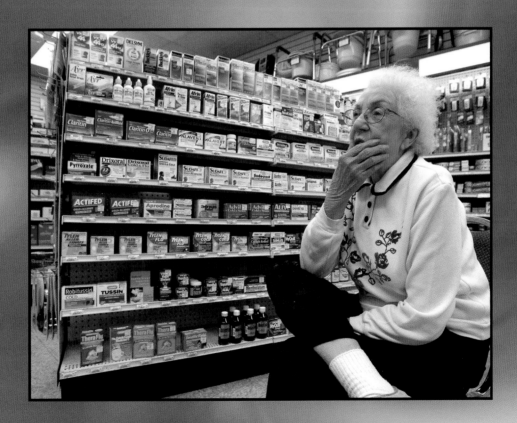

Hal Marcovitz

Produced by OTTN Publishing, Stockton, New Jersey

Mason Crest Publishers
370 Reed Road
Broomall, PA 19008
www.masoncrest.com

3 5 7 9 8 6 4 2

Library of Congress Cataloging-in-Publication Data

Marcovitz, Hal.
   Issues in health care / Hal Marcovitz.
      p. cm. — (Gallup major trends and events)
   Includes bibliographical references and index.
   ISBN-13: 978-1-59084-964-4
   ISBN-10: 1-59084-964-7
   1. Medical care. 2. Medical policy. 3. Health care reform. I. Title. II. Series.
   RA393.M294 2006
   362.1—dc22
                          2005016746

TABLE OF CONTENTS

Introduction

By Alec Gallup, Chairman, The Gallup Poll

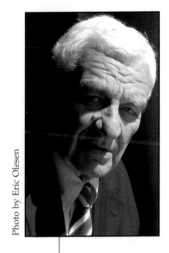

Photo by Eric Olesen

In ways both obvious and subtle, the United States of today differs significantly from the United States that existed at the turn of the 20th century. In 1900, for example, America had not yet taken its place among the world's most influential nations; today the United States stands by itself as the globe's lone superpower. The 1900 census counted about 76 million Americans, largely drawn from white European peoples such as the English, Irish, and Germans; 100 years later the U.S. population was approaching 300 million, and one in every eight residents was of Hispanic origin. In the first years of the 20th century, American society offered women few opportunities to pursue professional careers, and, in fact, women had not yet gained the right to vote. Though slavery had been abolished, black Americans 100 years ago continued to be treated as second-class citizens, particularly in the South, where the Jim Crow laws that would endure for another half-century kept the races separate and unequal.

The physical texture and the pace of American life, too, were much different 100 years ago—or, for that matter, even 50 years ago. Accelerating technological and scientific progress, a hallmark of modern times, has made possible a host of innovations that Americans today take for granted but that would have been unimaginable three generations ago—from brain scans to microwave ovens to cell phones, laptop computers, and the Internet.

No less important than the material, social, and political changes the United States has witnessed over the past century are the changes in American attitudes and perceptions. For example, the way Americans relate to their government and their fellow citizens, how they view marriage and child-rearing norms, where they set the boundary between society's responsibilities and the individual's rights and freedoms—all are key components of Americans' evolving understanding of their nation and its place in the world.

The books in this series examine important issues that have perennially concerned (and sometimes confounded) Americans since the turn of the 20th century. Each volume draws on an array of sources to provide vivid detail and historical context. But, as suggested by the series title, GALLUP MAJOR TRENDS AND EVENTS: THE PULSE OF OUR NATION, 1900 TO THE PRESENT, these books make particular use of the Gallup Organization's vast archive of polling data.

There is perhaps no better source for tracking and understanding American public opinion than Gallup, a name that has been synonymous with opinion polling for seven decades. Over the years, Gallup has elicited responses from more than 3.5 million people on more than 125,000 questions. In 1936 the organization, then known as the American Institute of Public Opinion, emerged into the spotlight when it correctly predicted that Franklin Roosevelt would be reelected president of the United States. This directly contradicted the well-respected Literary Digest Poll, which had announced that Alfred Landon, governor of Kansas, would not only become president but would win in a landslide. Since then Gallup polls have not simply been a fixture in election polling and analysis; they have also cast light on public opinion regarding a broad variety of social, economic, and cultural issues.

Polling results tend to be most noticed during political campaigns or in the wake of important events; during these times, polling provides snapshots of public opinion. This series, however, is more concerned with long-term attitude trends than with responses to breaking news. Thus data from many years of Gallup polls are used to trace the evolution of American attitudes. How, for example, have Americans historically viewed immigration? Did attitudes toward foreign newcomers shift during the Great Depression, after the 1941 Japanese attack on Pearl Harbor, or after the terrorist attacks of September 11, 2001? Do opinions on immigration vary across different age, gender, and ethnic groups?

Or, taking another particularly divisive issue treated in this series, what did Americans think about abortion during the many decades the procedure was generally illegal? How has public opinion changed since the Supreme Court's landmark 1973 *Roe v. Wade* decision? How many Americans now favor overturning *Roe*?

By understanding where we as a society have been, we can better understand where we are—and, sometimes, where we are going.

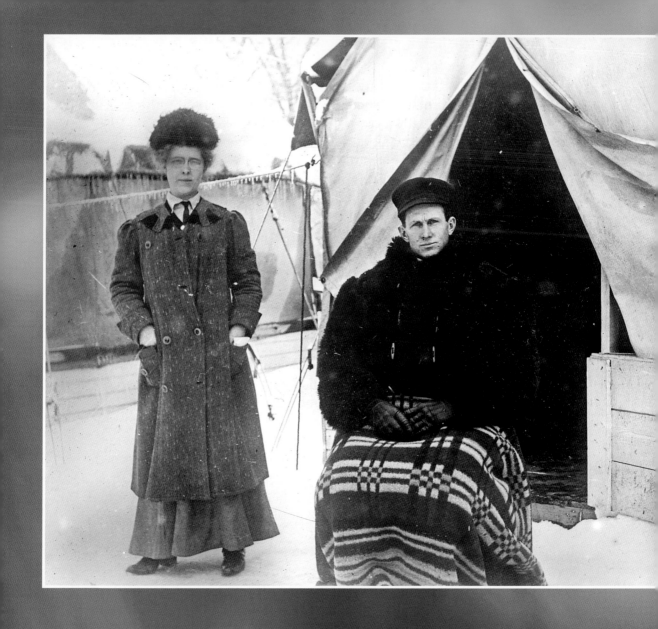

1 LIVING TO 100

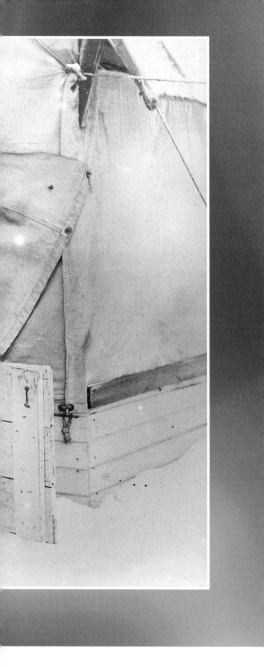

Quarantined victims of tuberculosis pose outside their tent. A century ago, tuberculosis was incurable and killed Americans at a rate of almost 20 per 10,000. Today, antibiotics have largely eradicated the disease from the United States.

A little more than a century ago, in 1900, the average life expectancy for an American citizen was 47. Many people lived well past that age, but untreatable diseases such as influenza, tuberculosis, and pneumonia caused innumerable premature deaths. Some diseases, such as diphtheria, measles, and whooping cough, took an especially devastating toll on children, dramatically driving down the average lifespan. In 1900 the infant mortality rate stood at 165 per 1,000 live births. In other words, for every thousand babies born alive, 165 would not survive to their first birthday.

As the 20th century proceeded, however, significant medical progress was made. During that time, for example, cures and vaccines were found for horrific diseases. Additionally, technological improvements helped doctors perform more accurate diagnoses and conduct surgeries that generations of past doctors never envisioned. Such progress proved tremendously beneficial for Americans. In 2000 the U.S. Census Bureau declared that life expectancy had reached 77 years—30 years had been gained since 1900. Infant mortality had shrunk to less than 7 per 1,000 live births—more than 23 times lower than the infant mortality rate a century earlier.

Disease statistics go a long way in telling the story. In 1900, for instance, tuberculosis caused nearly 20 deaths per 10,000 people; influenza was responsible for more than 20 additional deaths per 10,000, and pneumonia killed at about the same rate. Today, tuberculosis has been virtually wiped out. Similarly, while influenza and pneumonia are still very much a concern, the drugs developed to treat their symptoms have made them much less deadly. In 2001, for example, the U.S. National Center for Health Statistics reported that influenza and pneumonia accounted for just 2 deaths per 10,000 people—a fraction of the number they had killed a century ago.

Americans are today living longer than they ever have. In 2005 life expectancy for American males stood at nearly 75 years, while the typical female could expect to live past 80. Of course, many Americans live well beyond the average. People in their 90s, and even those reaching 100 years old or more, are increasingly common.

Living to See 100?

"Doctors say that, in the future, many more people will live to be 100 years old. How does the idea of living to be 100 seem to you—would you like to, or not?"

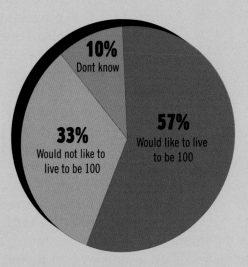

10%
Dont know

33%
Would not like to
live to be 100

57%
Would like to live
to be 100

Poll taken June–July 1950; 1,363 total respondents
Source: The Gallup Organization

KEEPING ACTIVE

At one time, the notion of such a lengthy life was not so attractive. The Gallup Organization, a national polling institute, has regularly gauged the opinion of Americans on the state of their own health. In the summer of 1950, a Gallup poll asked Americans this question: "How does the idea of living to be 100 seem to you—would you like to, or not?"Only 57 percent of the respondents said the idea was appealing.

This relative lack of enthusiasm for the idea of reaching age 100 may have had its roots in the belief that advanced age is always accompanied by painful and debilitating illnesses. But that isn't necessarily the case, especially today. In recent years, medical research has proven that people who keep themselves fit—who eat a nutritious diet, exercise, and don't smoke—can live long lives without the burden of illness. "People used to say, 'Who would want to be 100?'" commented Dr. Thomas Perls, a professor at Harvard University Medical School and director of the New England Centenarian Study, which studies the effects of aging on the human body. "Now, they're realizing it's an opportunity."

Scientists recently concluded that there is no reason that life expectancy can't be extended several more decades. This means that at some point—perhaps as soon as the year 2060—an average lifespan of 100 may be possible, at least in developed countries. In fact, researchers at the Faculty of Biology and Medicine of Switzerland's University of Lausanne made just that prediction in 2004.

In 2005 the U.S. Census Bureau reported that there were 50,000 people over the age of 100 (called centenarians) in the United States. Meanwhile, a United Nations projection estimates that by 2050 the number of centenarians in America could climb to nearly 300,000.

Of course, people engage in many behaviors that can cut their lives short. For instance, smoking remains

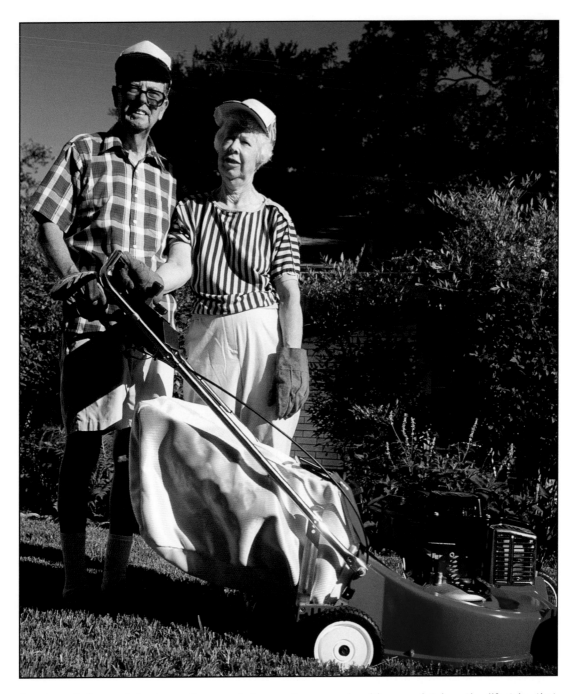

Americans today are living longer than ever before, and many senior citizens maintain active lifestyles that challenge long-held stereotypes.

a national habit, with one in four Americans admitting that they continue to light up—even after decades of warnings by public health officials and family doctors. Similarly, poor nutrition and overeating also can lead to debilitating illnesses. According to the National Center for Health Statistics, the leading causes of death for Americans in 2001 were heart disease, which claimed the lives of 85 out of 10,000 people, and cancer, which killed 19 per 10,000. Heart disease is directly related to smoking and overeating, while some forms of cancer are caused by smoking.

Still, Americans are not only living longer but also feeling better. The image of the white-whiskered grand-pa snoozing in a rocking chair may be familiar to Americans in contemporary society, but it is not necessarily true. Rather than snoozing and relaxing, many older Americans have elected to stay employed well past the traditional retirement age of 65. Tommy Peoples, an 82-year-old interviewed in 2005 by *Philadelphia Inquirer* reporter Michael Vitez, is a good example. When asked why he kept working after 63 years of employment with the same company, Peoples replied, "I think it keeps your brain active. You got to keep thinking." His secret to longevity? Exercise and a nutritious diet. Peoples swims three miles a week, drinks green tea, and snacks on carrots. "I don't do sugar at all," he said. "I haven't done sugar since the Army."

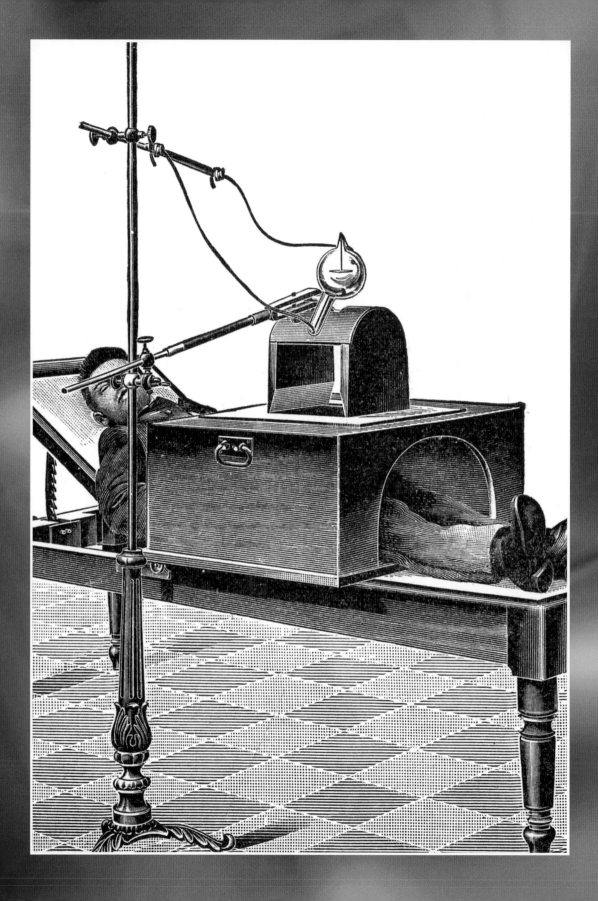

2

MEDICINE'S GREAT LEAP FORWARD

By the end of the 19th century, the world was on the verge of a great leap forward in scientific and technological knowledge. One facet of life that would greatly benefit from new discoveries and new technologies, along with the application of greater resources, was medical care.

As early as 1864, French chemist Louis Pasteur had discovered that germs cause disease and that people could spread germs by simply touching one another. Later, British physician Joseph Lister would advocate sterilization of medical instruments to cleanse them of germs. The germ theory of disease gained acceptance only gradually within the medical community, but in 1876 Lister visited America and urged physicians to sterilize their instruments. By the 1890s, most American surgeons were following his advice.

In 1895 the German scientist Wilhelm Roentgen made another discovery that would revolutionize medical diagnosis. Quite by accident, Roentgen found that a screen coated with barium glowed when it was struck by cathode

(Opposite) This 1895 woodcut depicts a patient in an early X-ray machine. Such machines were in use a mere six months after the discovery of X rays by the German physicist Wilhelm Roentgen.

rays emitted from an electrically charged tube—even when the tube was covered by cardboard. Roentgen deduced that the tube emitted an invisible radiation he called X rays. When Roentgen placed his hand in the path of the X rays, he was shocked to see the image of his bones underneath his skin. Roentgen immediately recognized the value of X rays to medicine. Within six months of his discovery, X-ray machines were arriving in hospitals, where they helped physicians diagnose broken bones, cancer, and other diseases and ailments.

Advances made by Pasteur, Lister, Roentgen, and others made possible better medical care, but the delivery of that care remained erratic. Insufficient doctors and hospitals were available to tend to the needs of the millions of immigrants living in the crowded tenements of America's teeming cities, where sanitation was lacking and disease spread quickly. Similarly, medical care was sparse in many rural areas and in the vast spaces of the West.

But shortcomings in the capacity of the nation's health system began to be addressed in the first decades of the 20th century. In 1870, for example, a mere 100 hospitals were in operation in all of the United States; by 1920 there would be 6,000. Most of the new hospitals were built by religious groups and other charitable organizations, although some labor unions sponsored the construction of hospitals and clinics for members and their families. With more hospitals, there was a need for more doctors and nurses. In 1870 Bellevue Hospital in New York established the first nursing school in the United States. By 1900 more than 400 nursing academies were in operation.

As for medical schools, in 1910 the American Medical Association and the Association of American Medical Colleges adopted tough standards for accreditation, designed to shut down disreputable schools that granted medical degrees overzealously. Meanwhile, universities also saw the need to establish pharmacy schools. In 1870 there were just 13 in operation in America; by 1900 there were 50.

PURE FOOD AND DRUGS

Another significant improvement in the nation's public health system occurred in 1906, when Congress passed the U.S. Pure Food and Drug Act. The law was adopted in the wake of the publication of *The Jungle*, a book by social reformer Upton Sinclair that exposed unsanitary conditions in the American meatpacking industry. Aside from addressing food processing, the law also required the manufacturers of patent medicines to list their ingredients on the labels. Until then, medicines were cheap and readily available through newspaper advertisements or door-to-door salesmen, and their manufacturers promised remedies for all manner of ailments—from headaches to diarrhea to teething pain. Many of these medicines included habit-forming opiates, which until then were unregulated and largely legal.

The Pure Food and Drug Act of 1906 led to the demise of the patent medicine trade. Eventually, amendments to the act required that drug ingredients meet standards of purity that the fly-by-night tonic and elixir makers couldn't possibly achieve. Meanwhile, the federal government as well as the state legislatures adopted statutes outlawing the use of opium and other narcotics.

Further medical needs became apparent when the United States entered World War I in 1917. The huge number of casualties prompted physicians to develop quick ways to deliver blood transfusions on the battlefield. Researchers found they could preserve blood through the addition of sodium citrate and by refrigerating their supplies. As a result, person-to-person battlefield transfusions were no longer necessary; instead, blood could be collected before a battle and refrigerated until it was needed. Some 126,000 Americans were

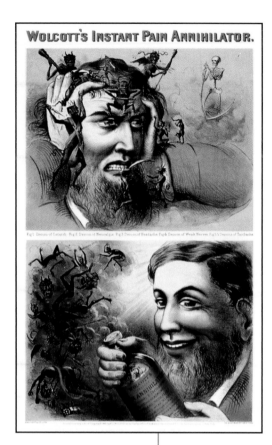

WOLCOTT'S INSTANT PAIN ANNIHILATOR.

Before the Pure Food and Drug Act of 1906, manufacturers of patent medicines like "Wolcott's Instant Pain Annihilator" made outrageous claims about their curative properties. Though some of these elixirs were essentially harmless, others contained highly addictive opiates.

killed in combat or died from disease during the conflict, and another 234,000 suffered battlefield wounds. When the war ended in November 1918, American servicemen began returning to friendly shores. Sadly, many who had survived the artillery shells, machine gun fire, and poison gas on the battlefield would find death awaiting them at home.

THE INFLUENZA PANDEMIC OF 1918

The first American case in what would become the world's worst flu pandemic (an epidemic covering an exceptionally large area) was reported at Fort Riley, Kansas, on March 11, 1918, when a young soldier reported to the post hospital complaining of a fever, sore throat, and headache. A second soldier soon arrived at the hospital with similar symptoms. By noon, 100 soldiers had been admitted, all of them in very ill health. Whether the outbreak started in Kansas or in the trenches of France has never been definitively established, but by the time the disease subsided, the influenza pandemic of 1918 would be responsible for at least 20 million deaths worldwide, including 600,000 in the United States.

Three waves of the flu swept through America before finally subsiding: the first wave arrived in the spring of 1918; the second in the fall, as infected servicemen started returning from Europe; and the third occurred in December, when a number of new deaths were reported after authorities believed the flu had run its course. Germs from the disease—called Spanish flu because of the erroneous belief that the outbreak had originated in Spain—were spread through the air by infected people speaking, sneezing, and coughing. The symptoms were unlike those of any other flu strain doctors had seen: a victim's skin would turn a bluish hue, often accompanied by purple blisters; there would be difficulty breathing as well as a hoarse, hacking cough producing a bloody sputum. Some people woke up in the morning and felt fine, but were dead by nightfall.

Soldiers training for deployment to Europe were hit hard by the disease. Army doctor Victor Vaughan, former president of the American Medical Association, recalled the scene when he arrived at Camp Devens outside Boston in September 1918:

> The saddest part of my life was when I witnessed the hundreds of deaths of the soldiers in the Army camps and did not know what to do. At that moment I decided never again to prate [boast] about the great achievements of medical science and to humbly admit our dense ignorance in this case. . . . I saw hundreds of young stalwart men in uniform coming into the wards of the hospital. Every bed was full, yet others crowded in. The faces wore a bluish cast; a cough brought up the blood-stained sputum.

The disease hit young and otherwise healthy adults the hardest—unlike most influenza outbreaks before and since, in which the very young and the elderly are most susceptible. Wrote Dr. Vaughn: "This infection, like war, kills the young, vigorous, robust adults. . . . The husky male either made a speedy and rather abrupt recovery or was likely to die." One of the flu sufferers was President Woodrow Wilson, who coughed and sneezed his way through the negotiations at the Treaty of Versailles, which officially ended World War I.

Finding the cause and the cure eluded physicians. Since Boston suffered many casualties, with more than a thousand victims, it was rumored that German spies had seeded Boston Harbor with influenza germs. "It would be quite easy for one of these German agents to

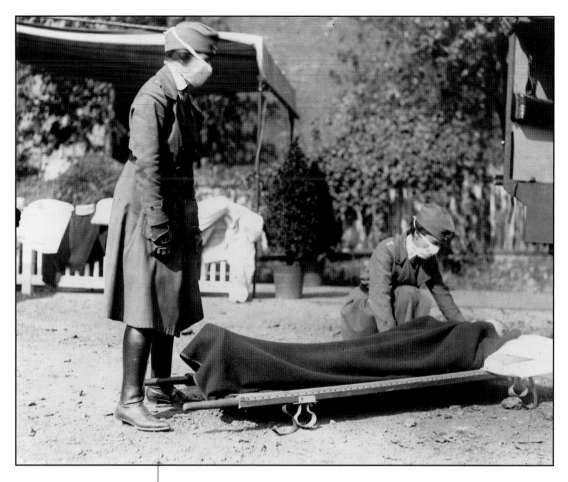

Wearing gauze masks to reduce the chances of infection, Red Cross nurses in Washington, D.C., observe a stretcher-bound influenza patient. The flu pandemic of 1918 claimed up to 600,000 lives in the United States alone.

turn loose influenza germs in a theater or some other place where large numbers of persons are assembled," said Lieutenant Colonel Philip Doane, an army sanitation expert. "The Germans have started epidemics in Europe," he asserted, "and there is no reason why they should be particularly gentle with America." However, Doane's suspicions were soon dismissed by public health officials. Another theory suggested that toxic vapors from the battlefields infected soldiers with flu-like symptoms. Others speculated that the flu was spread by dogs and cats.

Without knowing what caused the flu, medical researchers were unable to develop a vaccine to prevent its spread. In the meantime, public health officials urged people to wear gauze masks. Those who ventured outside without the masks risked arrest. In San Francisco, where thousands were infected during the second wave, people heard this rhyme repeated over the radio: "Obey the laws, and wear the gauze. Protect your jaws from septic paws." Nevertheless, some 23,000 San Franciscans contracted flu that fall; 2,122 died.

Other cities suffered as well. In Philadelphia, some 200,000 people attended a huge rally in late September to support a war-bonds drive. Just days after the rally, nearly 700 people reported flu symptoms. That fall, so many Philadelphians fell victim to the disease that the city's mortuaries ran out of coffins, and bodies were left in the streets. By the end of 1918, some 13,000 Philadelphians had lost their lives to the flu.

As he surveyed the ever-increasing death toll, Dr. Vaughan lamented, "If the epidemic continues its mathematical rate of acceleration, civilization could easily disappear from the face of the earth within a few weeks." But the influenza pandemic did not continue its mathematical rate of acceleration. Just as suddenly as it appeared, the flu went away. Medical researchers believe the flu simply ran out of victims who were susceptible to the virus.

Each year the flu claims thousands of American lives (in 2001, for example, the U.S. Public Health Service reported the death rate from flu and pneumonia at about 2 per 10,000). Most of these victims are elderly or very young, or they have immune systems that are already compromised. Today doctors have important weapons to fight influenza that were unavailable in

Woodrow Wilson was stricken with the flu while attending the Paris Peace Conference, but the 62-year-old president recovered. Unlike most strains of the virus, the so-called Spanish influenza of 1918 struck healthy young people the hardest.

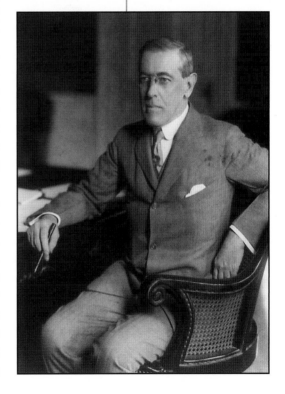

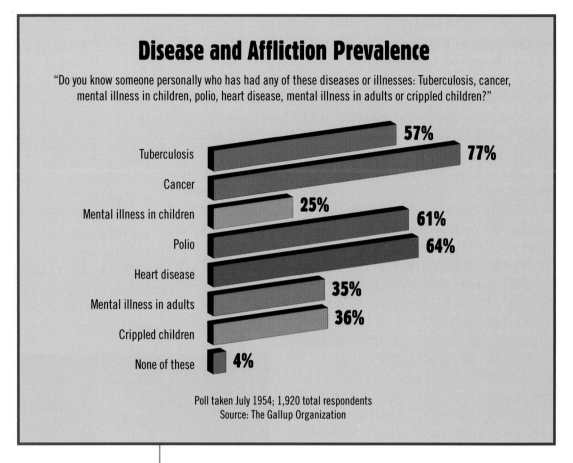

Disease and Affliction Prevalence

"Do you know someone personally who has had any of these diseases or illnesses: Tuberculosis, cancer, mental illness in children, polio, heart disease, mental illness in adults or crippled children?"

- Tuberculosis — **57%**
- Cancer — **77%**
- Mental illness in children — **25%**
- Polio — **61%**
- Heart disease — **64%**
- Mental illness in adults — **35%**
- Crippled children — **36%**
- None of these — **4%**

Poll taken July 1954; 1,920 total respondents
Source: The Gallup Organization

1918: vaccines to prevent infection (though there is no guarantee that the vaccine developed in a particular year will be effective against an influenza strain that emerges that year) and antiviral drugs to treat those who have been infected. While these advances have mitigated the effects of influenza, the primary reason the world has not suffered a repeat of 1918 is that a strain as lethal as the so-called Spanish flu has not emerged in the years since. But, many experts caution, it is only a matter of time before one does.

THE WHITE PLAGUE

Today tuberculosis causes far fewer deaths in the United States than does flu and pneumonia. According to Public Health Service statistics, in 2001 tuberculosis was responsible for death in just 1 out of every 300,000 Americans (although a rising occurrence of the disease in impoverished countries has raised alarms among health organizations worldwide).

Tuberculosis wasn't always so rare in the United States. In 1900 tuberculosis killed at a rate of 19 per 10,000 Americans. Worldwide, it has been estimated that for the 200 years between 1700 and 1900, tuberculosis was responsible for the deaths of no fewer than 1 billion people. As evidence of just how widespread the disease had become, in 1954, as the cure for tuberculosis was first being made available on a widespread basis, a Gallup poll reported that some 57 percent of Americans knew a tuberculosis victim. It seemed many people had a tuberculosis patient in their families or had friends who suffered from the disease.

Tuberculosis is caused by highly contagious bacteria spread from person to person through microscopic droplets expelled in a breath, sneeze, or cough. Many people contract tuberculosis but never manifest symptoms; in this condition, known as latent tuberculosis, the disease is kept in check by the body's immune system. In some cases in which the immune system has broken down—such as in a patient suffering from acquired immune deficiency syndrome (AIDS)—latent tuberculosis can become active. It is believed that a third of AIDS patients also are infected with latent tuberculosis.

Tuberculosis symptoms include coughing, fever, night sweats, and deterioration of the body. The lungs are affected the most, but the disease can also spread to the kidneys, brain, and bones. Tuberculosis patients suffer from persistent coughs and chest pain, and they often cough up blood. In many cases, the body becomes so ravaged by the disease and so weak that death becomes inevitable.

For centuries, no one knew how to cure the disease, which was known by various names, including "wasting disease," "consumption," and the "white plague," a term that did not refer to the racial composition of its victims but rather was a way to differentiate the disease from another great killer known to mankind, the bubonic plague, known as the "black death." A breakthrough in tuberculosis research finally came in 1882, when German physician Robert Koch discovered the bacterium that causes the disease, *Mycobacterium tuberculosis*. In a speech announcing his discovery, Koch said, "If the importance of a disease for mankind is measured by the number of fatalities it causes, then tuberculosis must be considered much more important than those most feared infectious diseases, plague, cholera and the like. One in seven of all human beings dies from tuberculosis. If one only considers the productive middle-age groups, tuberculosis carries away one-third, and often more."

With the cause of tuberculosis identified, medical researchers hunted for a cure. It would be a long time coming, however. Other discoveries would come first, but some of these supplied important information that would eventually lead to a cure for the white plague.

In 1910, for instance, German scientist Paul Ehrlich made a significant discovery. He found a chemical that killed the bacterium that causes the venereal disease syphilis. It was an important breakthrough, not only for syphilis sufferers but also because it showed that an outside substance could be introduced into the human body to wipe out invading bacteria. The concept could be applied to curing tuberculosis.

Eighteen years after Ehrlich's discovery, British researcher Alexander Fleming discovered that mold growing

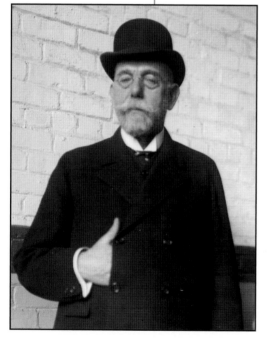

Dr. Robert Koch of Germany discovered the bacterium responsible for tuberculosis.

in a culture dish in his laboratory was effective in killing the bacteria also growing in the dish. The revelation led to the development of penicillin, which proved to be one of the most effective antibiotics ever discovered. Penicillin would help sufferers of pneumonia, scarlet fever, gonorrhea, and many other ailments, but it proved ineffective against tuberculosis. The research continued.

TAKING THE CURE

In the meantime, tuberculosis sufferers desperately searched for cures and methods to control their symptoms. At first, it was believed that warm climates could ease their suffering. Wealthy patients traveled to temperate regions, where they hoped relaxation and sunshine would provide a cure. While a therapy of warmth and sunshine may have provided tuberculosis sufferers some comfort, it did not cure the disease.

In 1873 New York physician Edward Livingston Trudeau contracted tuberculosis, which also had killed his brother. As Trudeau's health deteriorated, he resolved to spend the final months of his life at a hunting lodge in New York State's chilly Adirondack Mountains, where he had enjoyed many happy times. After an exhausting trip to the lodge, Trudeau arrived weak and wasted, expecting to die shortly. Instead, however, he felt himself grow stronger, invigorated by the fresh and cool mountain air. Trudeau soon established a sanatorium for tuberculosis sufferers at Saranac Lake, New York. The facility gained an international reputation; approximately 15,000 tuberculosis sufferers eventually would make the trek to Saranac Lake to "take the cure." Among them were author Robert Louis Stevenson, baseball player Christy Mathewson, and Manuel Quezon, president of the Philippines. In "The White Plague," an article published in *American Heritage* magazine, Elizabeth C. Mooney, the daughter of a Saranac tuberculosis patient, wrote:

Every train arriving in Saranac poured more TB victims into the village, anxious to try the wonderful mountain air and regain their shattered health. It was a village with one industry, a mecca for the dying, a source of new hope for many who had heard of the famous doctor's own miraculous cure. The local residents, hastily dusting off their spare bedrooms and stocking up on sputum cups and thermometers, rejoiced. The mountain air was their natural heritage, and their cash registers were jingling.

Trudeau's sanatorium featured wide outdoor porches, where the tuberculosis sufferers reclined overnight in "cure chairs." Trudeau believed that the cool mountain air could rejuvenate their lungs, and he urged patients to spend as much time as possible outdoors, even to spend cold winter nights swaddled in blankets on the porches. The patients also were made to rest for long periods.

Unfortunately, the cure did not work for everyone. Many people died at Saranac as well as at similar mountaintop treatment centers elsewhere in America. Trudeau also established a research center at Saranac, where he hoped to find a biological cure for the disease, but that solution would be found elsewhere.

Research was taking place at Rutgers University in New Jersey. There microbiologist Selman Waksman, an immigrant from the Ukraine, headed a team that was building on the discoveries of Fleming and Ehrlich, searching for a microorganism that would attack deadly bacteria. Waksman and his staff were intrigued by the fact that decomposing corpses did not infect the surrounding soil; instead, the scientists realized, something in the soil killed the bacteria in the corpses. "The remedies are in our own backyards," Waksman said.

The researchers experimented with many microorganisms found in soil, but they all proved to be worthless in fighting disease. Finally, in 1943, a farmer showed up at Rutgers with a sick chicken, hoping professors in the agriculture school could find a cure. After taking a culture from the chicken's gizzard, an alert biologist found a microorganism that he thought Waksman might be interested in. He sent the sample to Waksman's lab across campus, where Waksman's team grew it in a culture dish and found it to be similar to another microorganism they harvested from a sample of heavily manured soil. This time, both cultures proved effective in killing germs from many diseases — including tuberculosis. Their discovery led to the development of the drug streptomycin, which was first administered to a tuberculosis patient in 1944 and, miraculously, cured her symptoms. Although it took nearly a decade for the drug therapy to be refined and made widely available to tuberculosis patients, the cure had been found.

Unfortunately, millions of people died from tuberculosis before the drug became available. Author Elizabeth C. Mooney's mother was one such victim. She died in 1937, seven years before Waksman's discovery. For years, Mooney's mother had made regular visits to Saranac, hoping the chilly air would cleanse her tortured lungs. Arriving at her parents' home, Mooney recalled encountering her distraught father:

> "I couldn't help her," said my heartbroken father, taking my hand in his. I told him he managed to extend her life for seventeen years.
>
> It comforted him then. I wonder now whether what he did for her made any difference at all.

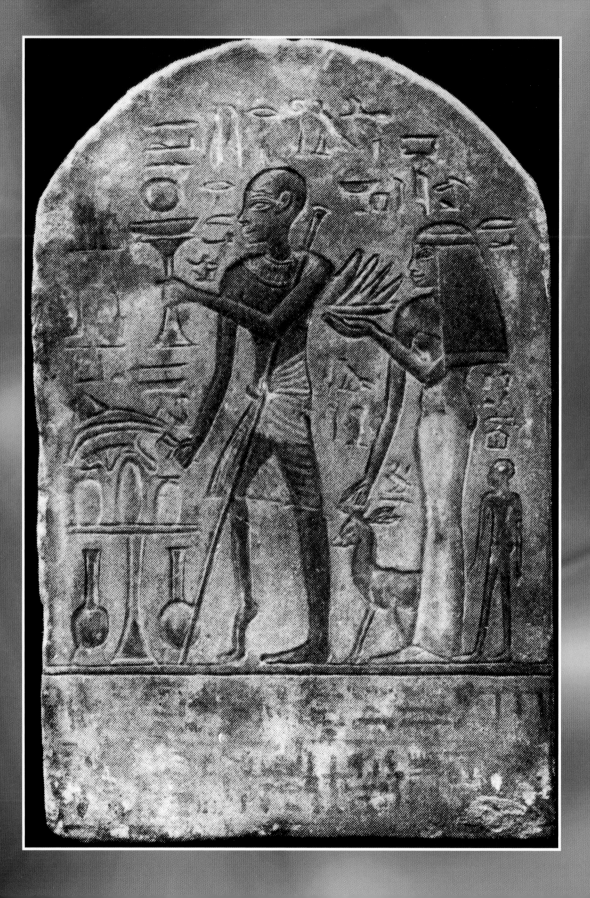

3

CONQUERING POLIO, CONFRONTING AIDS

Throughout the first half of the 20th century, polio victims suffered from a disease just as debilitating as tuberculosis. Although the death toll from polio never reached the proportions associated with tuberculosis, polio epidemics nevertheless arrived in waves and were concentrated in specific areas. In 1916, for example, a polio outbreak swept through America's Northeast, victimizing 28 out of every 100,000 people. New York City reported 9,000 victims that year, including some 2,400 fatal cases. As reported in Gerald N. Grob's *The Deadly Truth*, that summer a social worker told an interviewer that despite the boiling hot weather,

> mothers are so afraid that most of them will not even let the children enter the streets, and some will not even have a window open. In one house the only window was not only shut, but the cracks were stuffed with rags so that "the disease" could not come in. . . . I do not wonder they are afraid. I went to see one family about 4 p.m. Friday. The baby was not well and the doctor was coming. When I returned Monday morning there were three little hearses before

(Opposite) Polio has afflicted humanity since ancient times. In this Egyptian stela dating to around 1500 B.C., the man with a walking stick has a withered leg that almost certainly resulted from polio.

the door; all her children had been swept away in that short time.

The disease, officially known as poliomyelitis, is a highly contagious viral infection spread from human to human. It enters the mouth and intestinal tract, where it produces mild flu-like symptoms, such as sore throat, low fever, headache, and weariness. In most cases, the victim's antibodies can fight off the infection and, after a few days, the symptoms are eradicated. But if the body can't shake the virus, polio can spread to the spinal cord, brain, and central nervous system. Polio destroys cells in the spine and central nervous system, which can lead to paralysis.

Polio also can attack muscles used in breathing. When this happened to victims in the 1900s, they often died or were forced to live much of their lives sealed in a tank respirator, more familiarly known as an "iron lung"—a huge steel tube, the size of a small car, that used the force of air pressure to help the victim inhale and exhale. The first iron lung, which changed air pressure in the tank with two electric vacuum cleaners, was developed in 1927 by two physicians at Harvard University. Eventually, the machines were designed specifically for the purpose of manipulating chest muscles. They were by no means inexpensive. In the 1930s an iron lung cost $1,500—about the average price of a home at that time.

Engineers developed other contraptions they hoped would be effective in combating the effects of polio. One device, known as the rocking bed, tipped the patient up and down so that gravity would push air in and out of the lungs. The patient would be strapped into the bed, which was balanced on a central axis. When the bed was tipped forward, the patient's head would rise while his feet would fall, an action that would force air into the lungs. Tipped back, the patient's feet would rise and his head would fall, forcing air out. Another remedy called for the patient's chest to be wrapped in heated rolls of wool, under the theory that sudden heat followed by sudden cold would force the muscles to expand and contract.

Many polio victims fortunate enough to escape life in an iron lung and able to get by without using the other innovations of the era nevertheless found themselves suffering from some degree of paralysis, which often confined them to wheelchairs. The most famous victim of polio was President Franklin D. Roosevelt, who contracted the disease in 1921. Later, Roosevelt was elected to an unprecedented four terms as president. He didn't allow photographs of himself strapped in his wheelchair to be published, for fear that the American people would lose confidence in him if they knew of his handicap.

Because polio is contagious and people feared its spread as much as they feared the spread of tuberculosis, homes of polio victims often were quarantined. During epidemics, public places such as theaters and swimming pools were shut down. Doctors and nurses feared contracting the disease as much as anyone else. In 1934, during a polio epidemic in Los Angeles, 5 percent of the doctors and 11 percent of the nurses who treated polio patients came down with the disease themselves.

"Polio is a very visual disease," said historian David M. Oshinsky, author of *Polio: An American Story*. "You go into a restaurant, you don't know who has cancer or heart disease. But with polio, it's iron lungs and crutches and leg braces. It's the

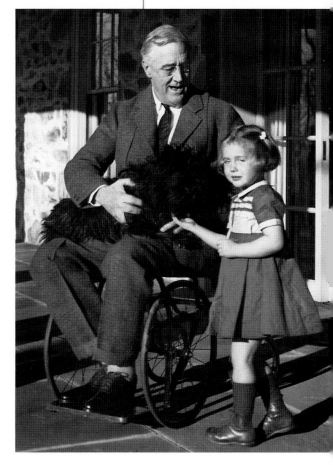

President Franklin D. Roosevelt, pictured here with his dog and a young friend, contracted poliomyelitis at age 39.

closing of swimming pools and movie theaters, and box scores in newspapers about [how many people] are getting it."

Dan Wilson, a Pennsylvania man who contracted the disease in the 1950s, recalled how his polio was diagnosed when he was five years old. "One of the tests was whether you could lift your head off the bed," he told reporter Marilyn Marchione for her 2005 article "Conquering the Killers." "I remember not being able to do that, and wondering what that meant."

In 1952 a record 57,628 new cases of polio were reported in the United States. Children were most susceptible to polio—originally, the disease was known as "infantile paralysis"—but adults were not immune (in 1954, for example, 35 percent of all polio victims were adults). A Gallup poll taken in 1954 reflected the depth of Americans' concern about polio. On a question asking respondents to name the most serious diseases or illnesses in the country, 44 percent listed polio; only two conditions were listed by a higher proportion of respondents: heart disease (including high blood pressure, strokes, and cardiovascular problems), named by 56 percent; and cancer, named by 71 percent. Another question from the same survey asked respondents to name the most serious diseases or illnesses facing children specifically, and the response was overwhelming: 85 percent listed polio; rheumatic fever, the next most frequently listed illness, was named by only 14 percent. Also, 61 percent of respondents said they knew a victim of polio.

USING POLIO TO DEFEAT POLIO

The microorganisms found to be effective against tuberculosis, syphilis, and other diseases failed to provide a cure for polio. And even today, there is no cure. Instead, researchers concentrated on developing a vaccine.

In 1955 University of Pittsburgh virologist Jonas Salk announced that he had used the poliovirus itself

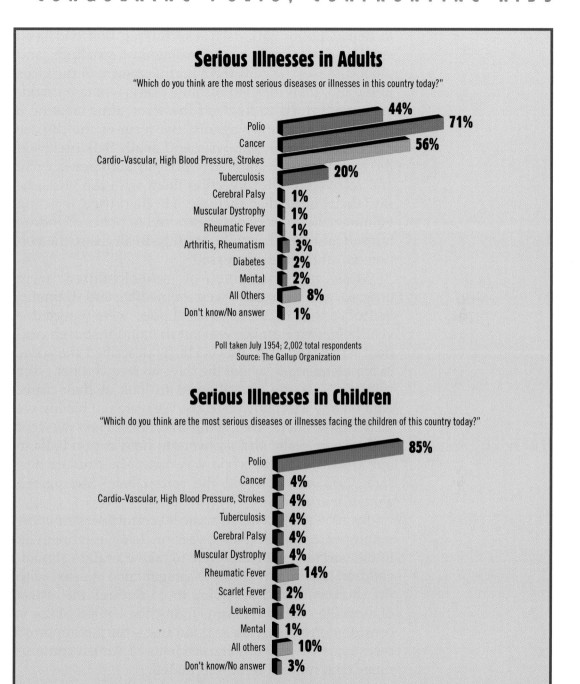

Serious Illnesses in Adults

"Which do you think are the most serious diseases or illnesses in this country today?"

Polio — 44%
Cancer — 71%
Cardio-Vascular, High Blood Pressure, Strokes — 56%
Tuberculosis — 20%
Cerebral Palsy — 1%
Muscular Dystrophy — 1%
Rheumatic Fever — 1%
Arthritis, Rheumatism — 3%
Diabetes — 2%
Mental — 2%
All Others — 8%
Don't know/No answer — 1%

Poll taken July 1954; 2,002 total respondents
Source: The Gallup Organization

Serious Illnesses in Children

"Which do you think are the most serious diseases or illnesses facing the children of this country today?"

Polio — 85%
Cancer — 4%
Cardio-Vascular, High Blood Pressure, Strokes — 4%
Tuberculosis — 4%
Cerebral Palsy — 4%
Muscular Dystrophy — 4%
Rheumatic Fever — 14%
Scarlet Fever — 2%
Leukemia — 4%
Mental — 1%
All others — 10%
Don't know/No answer — 3%

Poll taken July 1954; 2,002 total respondents
Source: The Gallup Organization

to defeat polio. Salk used a technique that had been employed to create a vaccine against smallpox and other diseases: he cultured a harmless form of the virus in the lab, then injected it into a body, where antibodies were formed to fight off the virus, thus creating a permanent immunity against the form of the disease that caused illness, paralysis, and death. Salk first tried the technique on children who had contracted polio and recovered; after injecting them with the virus, he saw their antibodies increase. He then tried injecting volunteers who were never exposed to polio, including himself and members of his family. In all cases, the volunteers' antibodies increased.

Mass immunizations of schoolchildren were ordered, and the results were immediate and dramatic. In 1955, a total of 28,985 cases of polio were reported; a year later, that number was cut in half. Pittsburgh resident Israel Ronna A. Casar Harris described the scene in her elementary school the day she received her polio vaccine: "No one was allowed to look at their arms. And no one was allowed to cry. We were not babies; we were first-graders. We got our injections. Then we went back to our seats, and we were to hold cotton balls to our arms. When everyone was done, she [the teacher] said, 'You may take off the cotton ball.' She passed along the trash can."

By 1959 physicians in some 90 countries were inoculating citizens with Salk's vaccine. Later, a refinement to the vaccine enabled people to take it orally—schoolchildren lined up to swallow a sugar cube injected with the vaccine instead of having to go through the ordeal of a needle shot in the arm. Today, the United States is considered to be virtually polio-free—the last reported cases were in 1979 among residents of Amish communities who refused to be vaccinated.

In other countries, the disease has reemerged. Many of the afflicted nations are in Africa and at one time were considered polio-free. In Nigeria, for example, the

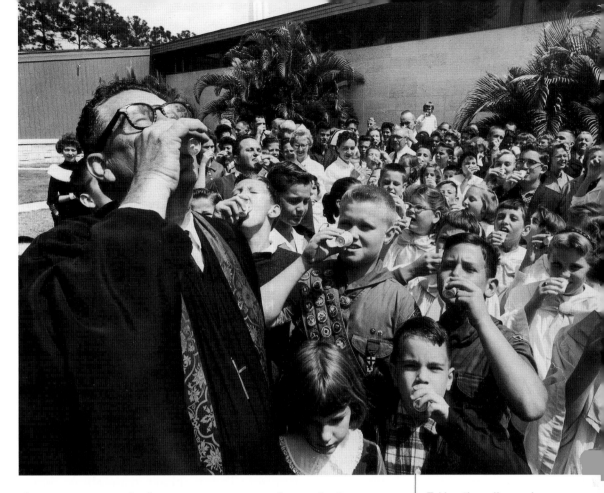

disease returned after rumors swept through the country that the polio vaccine caused sterility; this resulted in many people not getting vaccinated. International public health officials have tried hard to convince the Nigerians that the rumor is false. In 2004 officials from the United Nations persuaded Ibrahim Shekaru, the governor of the Nigerian state of Kano, to personally administer oral polio vaccines to several Nigerian children. "It's the beginning of the very final push to eradicate polio from Nigeria and the world," UN spokesman Gerrit Beger told a reporter. "Polio will have no hiding place any more from today."

THE SCIENCE OF THE HEART

The work of Jonas Salk, Selman Waksman, and other scientists proved that epidemics could be confronted and

Taking the polio vaccine orally, Florida, 1960. First developed by Jonas Salk, the polio vaccine has eradicated from the United States what had been one of the most feared childhood diseases.

defeated. Starting in the 1950s and 1960s, research in other fields resulted in further historic advancements in medical science. In 1959 the internal pacemaker was developed, providing heart patients with an artificial means to keep their hearts beating in a normal rhythm. In 1967 an even more dramatic advancement in the treatment of heart disease was accomplished by South African surgeon Christiaan Barnard, who performed the first human heart transplant. The operation on the patient, 53-year-old Lewis Washkansky, was regarded as a success, but the medications given to Washkansky to prevent his immune system from attacking the new heart also broke down his ability to fight off other infections. He died 18 days after the operation, a victim of double pneumonia. Nevertheless, Barnard's groundbreaking work showed that transplanting this most complicated and vital of human organs was possible. Soon other physicians would refine Barnard's techniques.

Shortly after Barnard performed the first heart transplant, 67 percent of respondents to a Gallup poll said they would be willing, upon their deaths, to be human heart donors. Today, heart transplants have become almost routine—in 2003, for example, 2,057 heart transplant operations were performed in the United States—and for most patients, the prognosis is good. According to the American Heart Association, the one-year survival rate for heart transplant patients is about 86 percent.

Clearly, though, there are not enough donor hearts to meet the needs of patients—some 50,000 people with failing hearts are on a waiting list for donor hearts. With so many people in need, some years ago many medical researchers asked the question: If a human heart could be transplanted, couldn't a heart be produced artificially and inserted into a human recipient? After all, other organs have been replaced by artificial devices. Patients with failing kidneys, for example, can be kept alive indefinitely through the process known as dialysis.

Organ Donation

"Would you be willing to have your heart or other vital organs donated
to medical science upon your death?"

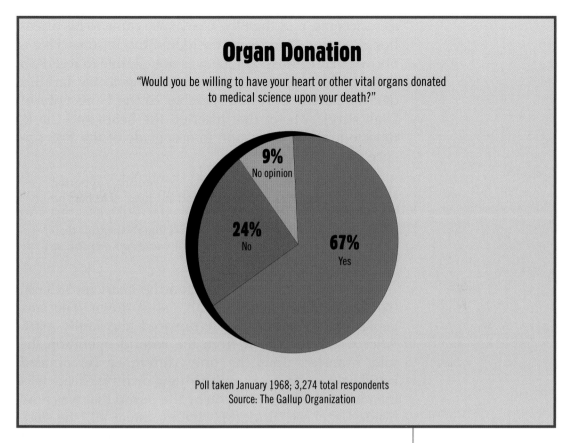

9%
No opinion

24%
No

67%
Yes

Poll taken January 1968; 3,274 total respondents
Source: The Gallup Organization

Developed in 1944, the dialysis machine does the work of the kidneys—it removes impurities from the patient's blood.

In 1969 an artificial heart—designed to pump blood when the patient's heart is too weak to perform adequately—was first implanted in a person. The patient, Haskell Karp of Skokie, Illinois, was kept alive on the artificial heart for three days until a donor heart could be found. Karp's transplant did not save his life; he died shortly after the operation. Still, the research has continued and refinements have been made.

In 1982 heart patient Barney Clark received an artificial heart designed by University of Utah medical researcher Robert Jarvik. Jarvik had been conducting trials of his artificial heart, the Jarvik-7, using monkeys as recipients, and then the Clark case came to his attention. Because Clark was considered too ill to survive a normal heart transplant, he was not eligible to receive a donated human heart. He was willing to try Jarvik's device. Donald Olsen, a member of the University of Utah surgical team that inserted the heart into Clark, reflected on the operation in a episode of the PBS science program *NOVA*:

> Here was a human being, alive, conversant, supported on a mechanical device. He had no heart. He had no conventional, traditional heart. And you know, the poets and writers have always said that the heart is really the center of love and personality and so forth and so forth. And he had none.

Shortly after doctors inserted the heart into Clark, the device failed when a valve shut down. The surgeons operated again and replaced the faulty part. After Clark recovered from the second operation, he told reporters that the only difference he noticed between his old heart and his new artificial heart was the mechanical sound made by the pump that was now inside his chest. "It doesn't bother me at all," he said. "Even when I'm awake it doesn't."

Barney Clark would live for just 112 days on his artificial heart. Clark's body never adapted to the radical surgery. He bled frequently, never regained his strength, and lived the final months of his life in a hospital room, virtually unable to move. Still, Jarvik and others continue working on an artificial heart. Since Clark's death, the Jarvik-7 has been implanted in 150 patients, and nearly two-thirds of them have survived long enough to receive a heart transplant.

Other researchers have concentrated on making artificial hearts smaller and less intrusive than the Jarvik-7, which had to be connected through a series of wires and tubes to a power unit the size of a refrigerator. In 2001, 59-year-old Robert Tools of Franklin, Kentucky, received a tiny artificial heart manufactured by Abiomed, a

Massachusetts company. Tools was suffering from congestive heart failure when his physician recommended him for the "AbioCor" heart. Unlike the heart implanted in Clark, the AbioCor is self-contained—the only external device needed to run the pump is a tiny battery pack that Tools could wear strapped to his waist. "The major obstacles to all artificial devices, and in particular the new technologies, are making sure the patients have adequate quality of life," said Dr. Mehmet Oz, a transplant authority. "The device needs to be forgettable. You need to have it on and live your life and not worry about it."

Tools died 156 days after the implantation of his heart. Doctors were encouraged, though, because they believed the main causes of his death were ailments not associated with the AbioCor. In addition to congestive heart failure, Tools suffered from diabetes and kidney disease. He died when his organs failed following severe abdominal bleeding. "Mr. Tools and his family members are heroes," said Dr. Robert Dowling, a member of the surgical team that implanted the AbioCor heart in Tools's chest. "Their willingness to be the first to participate in the AbioCor clinical trial could potentially pave the way for a revolutionary treatment option for advanced heart disease."

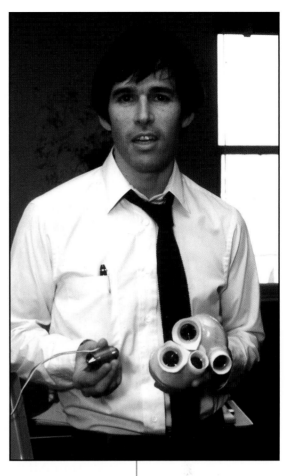

Dr. Robert Jarvik poses with the Jarvik-7, the artificial heart he created, 1981.

THE FIGHT AGAINST AIDS

In 1981 medical researchers recognized what was becoming an unusual and deadly trend: otherwise healthy homosexual men were contracting and dying from pneumonia and a rare form of cancer known as Kaposi's sarcoma. What made researchers believe the two diseases were linked was the fact that both ailments often were found in people with weakened immune systems. That year, 234 victims—mostly gay men—died from diseases mostly associated with weakened immunity. At first, the new syndrome was referred to as "gay-related immune disease," but researchers soon realized that a victim didn't have to be gay to be afflicted. Cases were reported among both men and women—particularly intravenous drug users and recipients of blood transfusions—regardless of their sexual orientations. The condition was then renamed acquired immune deficiency syndrome, or AIDS.

But what caused AIDS? That answer was provided in 1984 by French researchers, who established that AIDS is caused by a virus that attacks the immune system by destroying white blood cells—which help fend off disease and infection. Studies concluded that the virus, named human immuno-deficiency virus, or HIV, is transmitted by infected blood and semen.

Meanwhile, the death toll from AIDS had started rising. In 1982 a total of 853 people were known to have died from AIDS; a year later that figure stood at 2,304. In 1984 more than 11,000 cases were diagnosed, and the death toll hit 5,620. During the 1980s, a number of celebrities contracted AIDS. Actors Rock Hudson and Robert Reed, ballet dancer Rudolf Nureyev, and fashion designer Roy Halston joined the list of AIDS casualties. Professional tennis player Arthur Ashe succumbed to AIDS in 1993 after contracting the disease from a blood transfusion.

Early on, public health officials advised that most Americans didn't need to fear contracting AIDS; those at greatest risk were intravenous drug users who shared needles and people who engaged in casual sex without using condoms. Still, the public feared the

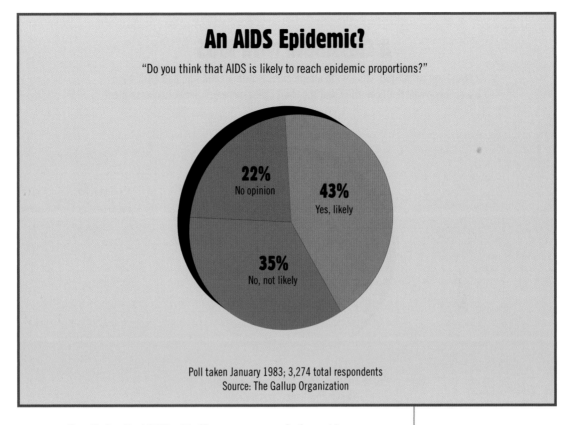

An AIDS Epidemic?

"Do you think that AIDS is likely to reach epidemic proportions?"

22%
No opinion

43%
Yes, likely

35%
No, not likely

Poll taken January 1983; 3,274 total respondents
Source: The Gallup Organization

worst. On July 7, 1983, Gallup reported that 43 percent of Americans surveyed believed AIDS was "likely to reach epidemic proportions." Wrote pollster George Gallup, "Despite the repeated statements of health authorities that for the vast majority of Americans there is little or no risk of falling victim to the disease AIDS, many U.S. adults fear the disease is likely to reach epidemic proportions and do not believe an immediate cure will be found."

Three years later, Surgeon General C. Everett Koop declared that condoms were the only effective way to prevent the spread of AIDS. He published the booklet *Understanding AIDS*; by 1988 more than 100 million copies had been distributed by the federal government.

Nevertheless, misconceptions and, in some cases, hysteria about the disease continued. In 1986, for

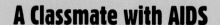

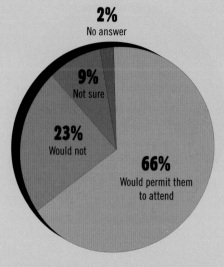

A Classmate with AIDS

Would you permit your children to attend classes with a child who had AIDS, even
if a county medical officer ruled that the child posed no health threat to classmates?

2%
No answer

9%
Not sure

23%
Would not

66%
Would permit them
to attend

Poll taken March 1986; 1,341 total respondents
Source: The Gallup Organization

example, 14-year-old hemophiliac Ryan White, who contracted AIDS from a contaminated blood transfusion, was barred by a court order from attending classes at his Indiana school. The injunction was lifted when a local health officer declared that Ryan posed no risk to his classmates. Ryan was permitted to return to school, but when he did so he found nearly half the seats empty. Parents of Ryan's classmates took their children out of school rather than risk exposing them to AIDS. A Gallup poll released on April 17, 1986, showed that many parents shared similar, albeit unfounded, concerns. The poll reported that 23 percent of parents in the United States would not let their children attend school with an HIV-positive classmate. Concluded pollster George Gallup Jr.:

The "at-risk" population almost exclusively comprises homosexual and bisexual men, intravenous drug users, people who receive blood transfusions from infected donors, and the sex partners and children of AIDS victims.

Public health officials note that although the spread of AIDS is rampant among the at-risk groups, its incidence outside these groups remains stable, at only 1% of reported cases. Nevertheless, there is considerable public concern that the disease may spread to the broader population.

Ryan White died in 1990. That year, he was one of 18,477 AIDS victims.

By 2003 an estimated 524,060 Americans had died from AIDS, according to the U.S. Centers for Disease Control and Prevention (CDC). Worldwide, AIDS was believed to have claimed more than 20 million victims,

Ryan White, a hemophiliac, developed AIDS after receiving an HIV-tainted blood transfusion. The Indiana teen's story drew national attention when school officials, fearing that other students would be infected, obtained an injunction barring him from attending classes— a reflection of the sort of ignorance that was common in the early years of the AIDS epidemic.

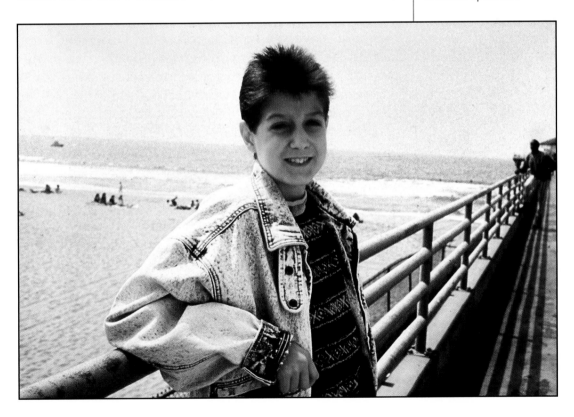

most of them in underdeveloped countries in Asia and Africa, by 2004. While no cure has been found and no vaccine has been developed, medical advances started bearing fruit in the 1990s, when drugs were discovered that could slow the disease's progression, assisting the body in fighting off infections. What's more, the extensive public information programs that urged people to practice safe sex also helped reduce the transmission of the disease. In June 2001 the CDC reported: "As a result of these and other HIV prevention efforts and increases in societal awareness of and response to the AIDS epidemic, new infections in the United States, which had risen rapidly to a peak of 150,000 per year in the mid-1980s, declined to an estimated 40,000 per year since 1992."

Still, the spread of AIDS remains a significant public health concern, especially in the gay male community. Indeed, according to the CDC, HIV infections among men who have sex with men rose by 11 percent from 2000 to 2003, while remaining stable in the rest of the general public. Another problem related to the disease was recognized in 2005, when public health officials in New York State discovered a new, highly aggressive and drug-resistant strain of HIV. Medical researchers have speculated that the disease has evolved, becoming more resistant to the drugs used for treatment. Once again, gay men who engage in unprotected sex — in particular, those who abuse a form of the drug methamphetamine known as "crystal meth," which relaxes inhibitions and leads to promiscuous behavior — are believed to be most at risk. The men who have contracted the new form of HIV are known to have engaged in casual, unprotected sexual relations with multiple partners. Gal Mayer, associate medical director of Callen-Lorde Community Health Center in New York, said in a February 2005 *Philadelphia Inquirer* article: "We're seeing new infections that already, one, two, three or four medications can't be used to treat."

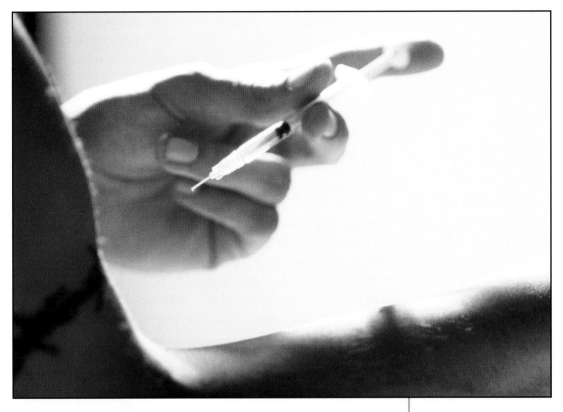

NEW THREATS TO HEALTH

In recent decades, new threats to the public health have continually surfaced. However, none has been as devastating as the flu pandemic of 1918, or the tuberculosis and polio epidemics, or AIDS.

Before 1977 very few people outside the general vicinity of Lyme, Connecticut, had heard of the tiny town. Soon the name would become well known, however, after children in the community started displaying the type of muscle aches and joint pain usually associated with arthritis—a very uncommon ailment for young people. Other symptoms included a skin rash, fever, fatigue, and headache. An investigation revealed that the children were afflicted with bacteria spread through the bite of a deer tick. By the 1980s people were told to be on guard against "Lyme disease." Health

In recent years, rates of new HIV infections have once again been rising among gay males. One reason, experts say, is widespread abuse of crystal meth, a drug that removes inhibitions and causes risky sexual behavior.

authorities advised that hikers and campers wear long sleeves and long pants, use insect repellent, and check their bodies frequently for ticks when in wooded or grassy areas.

Nevertheless, in 2002 more than 23,000 cases of Lyme disease were reported—and not just in Connecticut. In fact, Lyme disease has spread to the West Coast. A 2003 Gallup poll found 3 percent of people very worried about Lyme disease and 15 percent somewhat worried. For those who do become infected, antibiotic drugs are prescribed, and this treatment is usually effective.

Unlike Lyme disease, West Nile virus is spread by mosquitoes. Many people who contract West Nile virus never realize they are infected, but older people and others with weak immune systems develop flu-like symptoms. In more serious cases, victims contract

Deer ticks like these can transmit Lyme disease. Symptoms include joint and muscle aches, skin problems, headaches, and fever.

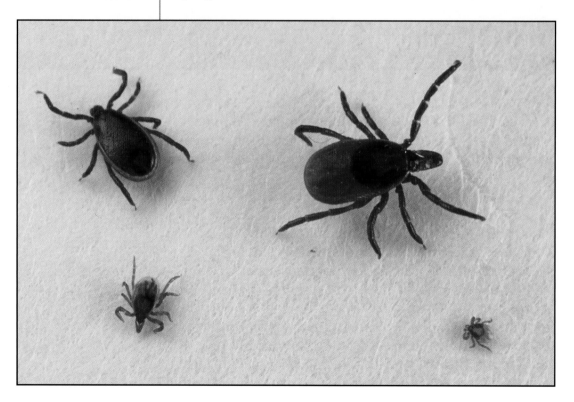

AMERICANS AND ALZHEIMER'S DISEASE

Shortly after President Ronald Reagan left the White House in 1989, he disclosed to the American people that he had been diagnosed with Alzheimer's disease. Reagan died in 2004 from complications of Alzheimer's.

The disease was first identified in 1907 by Dr. Alois Alzheimer, who discovered a physical deterioration in the brain cells of certain patients suffering from some forms of dementia (a loss of intellectual abilities). Alzheimer's disease afflicts older people, who over time lose their memories. As the disease progresses, patients stop recognizing family members, and many patients can't even remember who they are. Patients with Alzheimer's typically survive between 2 and 20 years after the disease is diagnosed. Eventually, their physical health also breaks down, although medical researchers are unsure why; there may be some association between brain impairment and the body's ability to recover from disease.

According to the American Academy of Neurology, some 5 million Americans suffered from Alzheimer's disease in 2003, though half were undiagnosed. Barring a cure, the academy estimates that 8 million Americans will be afflicted with Alzheimer's disease by 2030. By 2050 the disease may afflict as many as 14 million Americans.

There is no question that Americans are far more fearful of Alzheimer's disease than they were years ago. In 1997, when a Gallup poll asked Americans to rank their health concerns, Alzheimer's disease did not receive enough mentions to be ranked in the poll. That year, Americans listed AIDS, cancer, and heart disease as the ailments they feared most.

By 2003, as it became known that Ronald Reagan was approaching the end of his life, fear of Alzheimer's definitely had become a concern for Americans. In fact, 37 percent of respondents in a Gallup poll said they worried about contracting the disease. While cancer and heart disease were still of greater concern for more Americans, Alzheimer's had surpassed AIDS. Not surprisingly, older Americans were most concerned about contracting Alzheimer's. The poll found that 42 percent of respondents over the age of 50 were concerned about contracting the disease, while 34 percent of people under 50 were concerned.

And perhaps because of Reagan's experience, nearly 79 percent of Americans feel the president should be required to undergo an annual test for Alzheimer's disease, according to a 2004 Gallup poll.

encephalitis—a swelling of the brain, which is a potentially fatal condition that usually requires hospitalization. There is no cure for West Nile virus; doctors can only treat the symptoms.

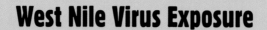

West Nile Virus Exposure

"How worried are you that you or someone in your family will be exposed to the West Nile Virus?"

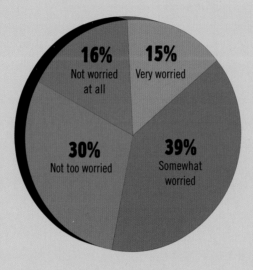

16%
Not worried
at all

15%
Very worried

30%
Not too worried

39%
Somewhat
worried

Poll taken September 2002; 1,010 total respondents
Source: The Gallup Organization

The first American cases of West Nile virus, which was originally identified in Egypt in 1937, occurred in the northeastern states in 1999. Since then the disease has been spreading west. To combat West Nile virus, most states have established eradication programs that use bacteriological agents to kill nests of mosquitoes; typically, stream banks and marshy areas are sprayed. In addition, homeowners are asked to make sure there are no stagnant pools of water on their properties—for example, in birdbaths, gutters, and wading pools—because these provide mosquitoes with ideal breeding grounds.

West Nile virus does not afflict as many people as Lyme disease—in 2004, for example, only 2,470 cases were reported. But West Nile virus can be deadly; 88 of the cases reported in 2004 were fatal. Perhaps because it can cause death, West Nile virus raises fears among the public. In 2002 a Gallup poll found 59 percent of women and 47 percent of men either very worried or somewhat worried about contracting the virus.

Severe acute respiratory syndrome (SARS), another viral disease that has raised public concern, originated in southern China in 2002. By early 2003, before the outbreak was contained, SARS had spread to some 25 countries in Asia, North America, South America, and Europe; the outbreak was contained by July. The disease—whose symptoms include high fever, headache, body aches, cough, difficulty breathing, and diarrhea—typically progresses to pneumonia. It is spread through close contact with an infected person, especially through coughing and sneezing. Of approximately 8,100 people stricken worldwide during the 2003 outbreak, 774 deaths were documented. Only eight people in the United States are known to have contracted the disease, and all had traveled to places with high rates of SARS infections, such as Hong Kong. Nevertheless, in 2003 Gallup polls showed an average of 37 percent of respondents harboring concerns about contracting SARS. One explanation may be that Toronto, Canada, was hit relatively hard by SARS, with 160 reported cases, including 16 fatalities. About 14 percent of Gallup respondents who had been planning to travel by air in 2003 said they changed their minds out of fear of contracting SARS.

In subsequent years, however, SARS did not reemerge as a global threat. Several cases were reported in China in 2004, but all were linked to laboratory research. Through the summer of 2005, there were no other documented cases.

FEAR OF BIOTERRORISM

Shortly after the terrorist attacks of September 11, 2001, Americans learned that terrorism could involve more

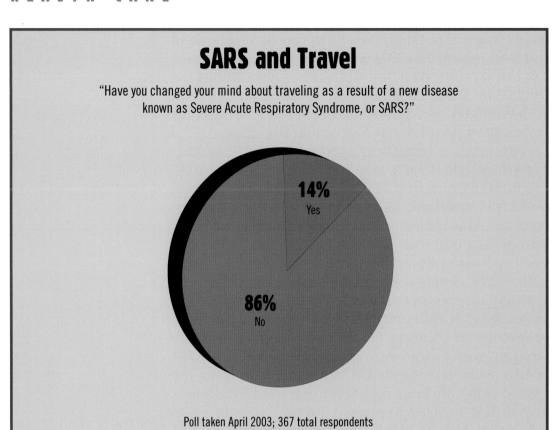

SARS and Travel

"Have you changed your mind about traveling as a result of a new disease known as Severe Acute Respiratory Syndrome, or SARS?"

14%
Yes

86%
No

Poll taken April 2003; 367 total respondents
Source: The Gallup Organization

than just hijacked airliners and suicide bombers. Only a few weeks after the attacks, Robert Stevens, the photo editor of a tabloid newspaper in Florida, contracted anthrax—a rare disease found mostly in farm animals but nevertheless deadly to humans. Cultured as spores, the disease can be spread through contact with infected skin or by inhalation. Anthrax sufferers develop skin rashes, high fevers, and flu-like symptoms. Anthrax can be fatal, but it also can be treated with antibiotic drugs, and most anthrax sufferers who receive treatment do recover.

Evidently, Stevens had come into contact with mail infected with anthrax spores. Over the next few weeks, anthrax-tainted envelopes were mailed to Tom Brokaw, an NBC news anchor, and Tom Daschle, the U.S. Senate majority leader. Neither man contracted the disease, as neither had handled the tainted letters. But one of Brokaw's assistants did come down with skin anthrax.

FBI agents determined that the mail in question had gone through a post office near Trenton, New Jersey, where some postal employees came into contact with the envelopes and contracted the disease. By the end of the year, 18 people had been infected with anthrax. Five of the victims, including Stevens and two of the postal workers, died from the disease. As of late 2005, authorities still hadn't apprehended the person or persons responsible for sending the anthrax-laced letters.

The deaths shocked Americans. In a November 2001 Gallup poll, bioterrorism emerged as the top health concern among respondents. Indeed, 22 percent of Americans named bioterrorism, anthrax, and smallpox the "most urgent health concern facing the country at this present time." Cancer and the cost of health care were tied for second, each with 19 percent, while AIDS was mentioned by 7 percent of respondents, and heart disease by 6 percent. According to the Gallup analysis:

> The power of public awareness is most obvious when current perceptions of the most urgent health problem (bioterrorism) are compared to another item on the list—heart disease. Heart disease is the leading cause of death in the United States, and affects millions of Americans, and yet no more than 7% of Gallup Poll respondents have ever mentioned it as the nation's most urgent health problem.

> To date, anthrax attacks within America have resulted in 18 confirmed cases of anthrax and tragically killed five people, but stories of anthrax have been very prominent in the news over the past several weeks. Combined with a general fear of terrorism following the attacks of Sept. 11, the public now views bioterrorism with a sense of urgency disproportionate to the total number of deaths it has caused.

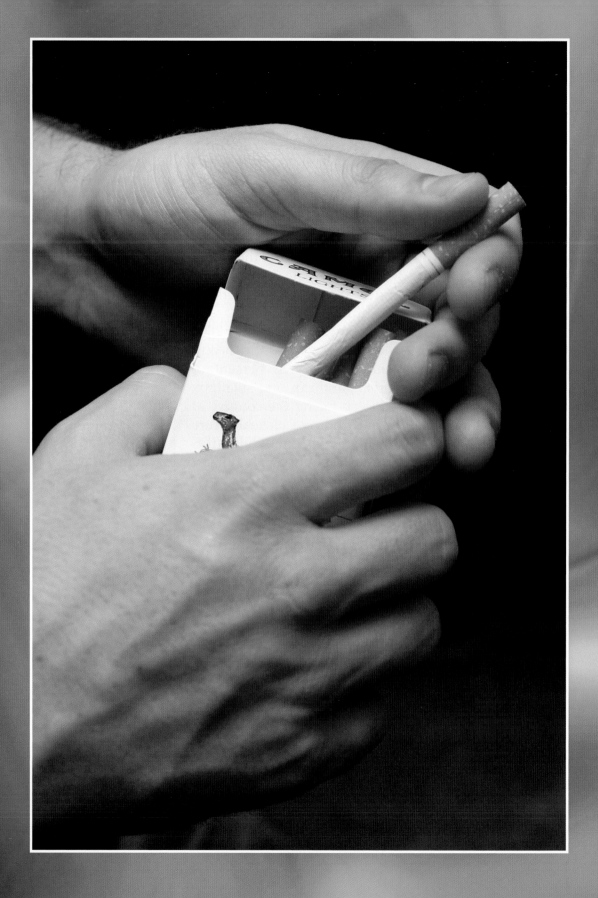

4

AMERICA'S CIGARETTE HABIT

Those watching the *Tonight Show* starring Johnny Carson on New Year's night in 1971 saw a bit of television history. At one minute before midnight, the Philip Morris tobacco company, manufacturer of Virginia Slims cigarettes, aired a commercial featuring a fashionable young woman proudly displaying her cigarette. It was a typical ad for the Virginia Slims brand, which is marketed to women. What made this particular ad so memorable, though, is that American viewers would never see another like it. The ad was the last cigarette commercial to air on American television.

The year before, an act of Congress prohibited cigarette advertising on television, effective January 2, 1971. The tobacco companies, which had fought the ban for two years, finally lost, but they had managed to convince Congress to begin the ban the day after New Year's. This would give them one final opportunity to reach the massive audiences watching college football's New Year's bowl games.

By the time Congress imposed its ad ban, the link between cigarette smoking and a host of

(Opposite) Despite the very well documented health risks associated with cigarettes, one in four Americans is a smoker.

health problems—including lung cancer, emphysema, and heart disease—was clear to American health officials and political leaders alike. Lawmakers singled out television for the ad ban not only because the medium reached virtually everyone in the United States but also because of the uniquely persuasive nature of TV.

Interestingly, the cigarette companies themselves were largely responsible for helping television become the influential source of news and entertainment it had become by the 1970s. During the early years of television, many large American corporations were hesitant to commit advertising dollars to the untested medium, yet the television networks found that tobacco companies were more than willing to sign on as sponsors. Some of television's earliest shows were underwritten by the tobacco industry. For example, Philip Morris was the first sponsor of *I Love Lucy*, an enormously popular situation comedy starring Lucille Ball and Desi Arnaz. To accommodate the sponsor, the producers were happy to have the stars play their scenes holding the company's cigarettes. *The Flintstones*, television's first prime-time animated sitcom, was sponsored by Winston cigarettes. The two main characters, cavemen Fred and Barney, ended the early shows by puffing on Winston cigarettes.

Cigarette companies also enlisted movie stars for their TV commercials. John Wayne, for example, starred in commercials for Camel cigarettes.

By the late 1960s, Congress—aiming to reduce America's cigarette habit—began debating restrictions on television advertising. With the passage of the 1970 law, there was optimism that such measures would eventually produce dramatic results. The TV ad ban remains in effect today, and many other restrictions on cigarette advertising have since been added, but the smoking habit continues to keep a firm hold on many Americans, thanks mostly to the addictive quality of nicotine, a major component of cigarette tobacco. Today an estimated 25 percent of the American population smokes cigarettes.

The fates of movie and television stars who helped sell cigarettes in the days before the TV ad ban attest to the dangers of smoking. Desi Arnaz died of lung cancer in 1986. Johnny Carson, who invariably had a cigarette burning in his ashtray on the *Tonight Show* set, died of emphysema in 2005. John Wayne fought lung cancer and heart disease for 16 years before losing his battle in 1979. Bea Benaderet, who supplied the voice of Betty Rubble on *The Flintstones*, died of lung cancer and emphysema in 1968. Jean Vander-Pyl, who did the voice of Wilma Flintstone on the show, died of lung cancer in 1999. VanderPyl's son, Michael O'Meara, recalled, "Everybody on the *Flintstones* smoked and all of them ended up dying of smoking-related diseases. . . . That little cute laugh that Betty and Wilma did with their mouths closed? They came up with that because when they normally laughed, because they were smokers, they coughed."

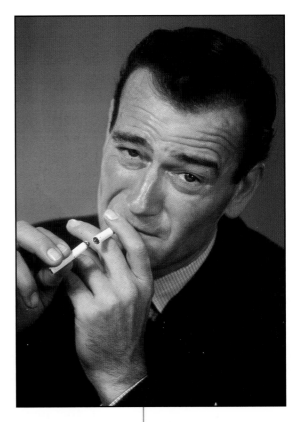

Movie star John Wayne appeared in TV commercials for Camel cigarettes. His tobacco habit ultimately proved fatal: Wayne succumbed to heart disease and lung cancer in 1979.

EVIDENCE OF ILL EFFECTS

A century ago, smoking cigarettes was one of the least common ways to use tobacco; pipe and cigar smoking, along with chewing tobacco, were much more popular among Americans. But early in the 1900s, chewing tobacco began to lose favor after public health agencies warned of the health hazards of spitting—it could help spread tuberculosis. Laws were established prohibiting spitting in the streets. Meanwhile, bars and restaurants stopped providing spittoons to their customers. With few places in public available to spit their wad of chewed tobacco, or chaw, many men gave up the habit.

In the meantime, technology was transforming American tobacco companies. Although cigarettes had been available for many years, the development of machines that could manufacture them quickly, using a thin, cheaply produced paper to hold the tobacco, helped the product gain a market. Also, the tobacco plantations developed a milder form of tobacco that could be inhaled. Tobacco used in cigars and pipes was too harsh to be drawn into the lungs; it made smokers cough.

From the start, some people were wary of cigarettes. In 1914, according to Edward M. Brecher's *Licit and Illicit Drugs*, Thomas A. Edison wrote that the cigarette "has a violent action in the nerve centers, producing degeneration of the cells of the brain, which is quite rapid among boys. Unlike most narcotics, this degeneration is permanent and uncontrollable. I employ no person who smokes cigarettes." Edison was wrong about the health effects—cigarette smoke does not destroy brain cells. Nevertheless, he was among the first people in science to be concerned about the health effects of smoking.

During the first decade of the 20th century, it was estimated that Americans smoked more than 4.2 billion cigarettes. By the end of the second decade, the popularity of cigarette smoking was primed to explode. World War I was a big part of the reason. Patriotic citizens, anxious to help Americans fighting in France, sent millions of free cigarettes overseas to be distributed to the troops. Indeed, the American Red Cross included packs of cigarettes in the parcels of food, letters, newspapers, and books it shipped to the men in the trenches. The result? Following the war, hundreds of thousands of men returned to their homes in America, and many of them were addicted to cigarettes.

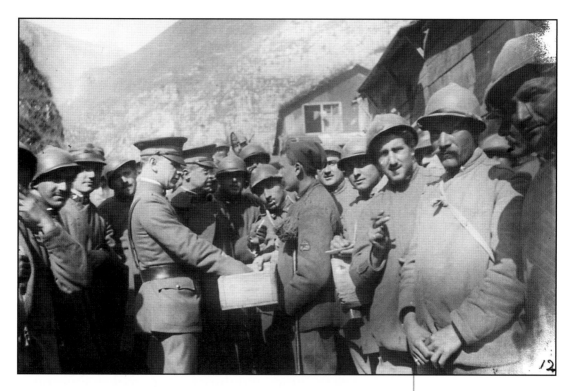

The Red Cross distributes donated cigarettes to American troops serving on the Italian front during World War I, 1918. After the war, thousands of soldiers returned home with cigarette habits.

Between 1910 and 1919, it was estimated that Americans smoked more than 24 billion cigarettes. During the following decade, that number rose dramatically, with Americans smoking no fewer than 80 billion cigarettes. By then, women were smoking as well. In 1924 Philip Morris introduced the Marlboro brand of cigarettes. Initially Marlboro was regarded as a woman's cigarette because of its blend of mild tobaccos. Only later would the company successfully market this cigarette to men as the choice smoke of the rugged, "Marlboro man" cowboy—another indication of the power of cigarette marketing.

With more people smoking, it didn't take long for the evidence of ill effects on their health to start mounting. For example, in 1927 a study in the British medical journal *Lancet* reported that almost every patient who died of lung cancer in England was a heavy cigarette smoker.

Nevertheless, by the 1950s Americans were smoking cigarettes in huge numbers. A Gallup poll reported in June 1957 that 42.5 percent of Americans—some 76 million people—smoked cigarettes. Seventeen percent said they had pack-a-day habits. That year, Dr. E. Cuyler Hammond of the American Medical Society and Dr. Daniel Horn of the American Cancer Society issued the first major warning about cigarette smoking, in a joint report titled *Smoking in Relation to Death Rates*. The paper concluded that cigarette smoking was a significant cause of lung cancer, chronic bronchitis, emphysema, and heart disease. In addition, the U.S. Public Health Service warned that there was "increasing and consistent evidence" that "excessive [cigarette] smoking is one of the causative factors of lung cancer."

Research into the deadly effects of smoking soon centered on the tar content of cigarette smoke. Each puff of cigarette smoke contains thousands of suspended particles that compose tar, a sticky brown substance that coats the lungs and throat of the smoker. Even people in the vicinity of smokers may suffer from what is known as "second-hand smoke," the smoke coming from others' cigarettes. Over the years it has been found that bystanders who regularly inhale second-hand smoke—such as the spouses or children of heavy smokers—may be affected. Tar contains some 4,000 chemicals, many of them cancer causing. Among its deadly chemicals are carbon monoxide, arsenic, benzopyrene, lead, ammonia, formaldehyde, cadmium, and cyanide.

Despite scientific evidence pointing to the hazards of cigarette smoke, many Americans during the late 1950s and early 1960s were unconvinced that cigarettes could be harmful. Indeed, a Gallup poll taken shortly after the Hammond and Horn report was made public revealed that only half the respondents believed cigarettes caused cancer; what's more, just 38 percent of smokers believed this. In addition, only 41 percent of Americans, including 32 percent of smokers, said they

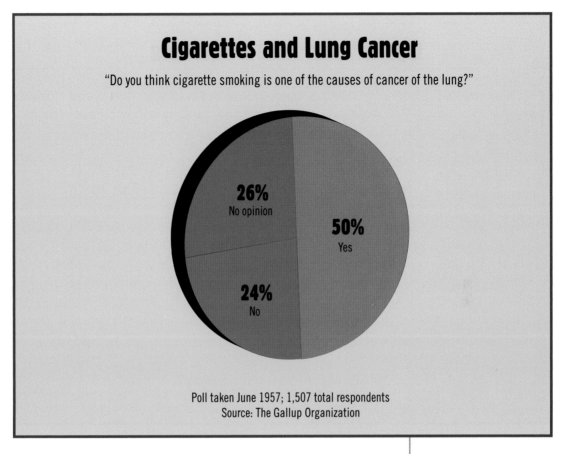

Cigarettes and Lung Cancer

"Do you think cigarette smoking is one of the causes of cancer of the lung?"

26%
No opinion

50%
Yes

24%
No

Poll taken June 1957; 1,507 total respondents
Source: The Gallup Organization

believed cigarettes caused heart disease. According to a July 1957 Public Opinion News Service release:

> Whether a person is disposed to believe that there is a cause-and-effect relationship between [cigarette] smoking and heart disease depends a great deal on his smoking habits, as was also true in the lung cancer survey results.
>
> In general, adults who smoke [cigarettes] are inclined to believe that there is no connection, while non-smokers believe there is.

The full weight of the federal government soon was put behind the evidence, however. On January 11, 1964, the Report of the Surgeon General's Advisory Committee on Smoking and Health was released. The

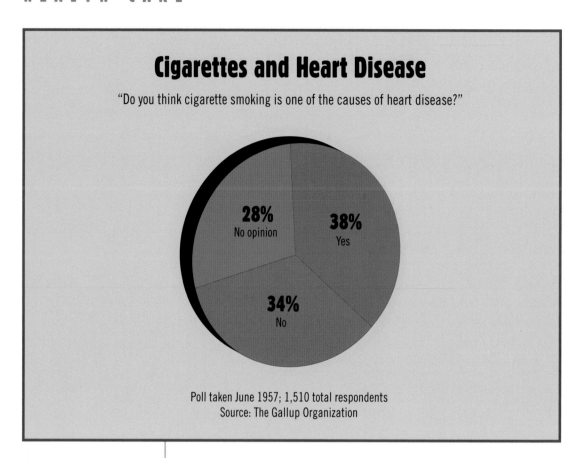

Cigarettes and Heart Disease

"Do you think cigarette smoking is one of the causes of heart disease?"

28%
No opinion

38%
Yes

34%
No

Poll taken June 1957; 1,510 total respondents
Source: The Gallup Organization

report stated, in no uncertain terms, that cigarette smoking shortens life and causes lung cancer, emphysema, bronchitis, and heart disease. This report seemed to have far more of an impact on smokers than the 1957 Hammond and Horn report. Within a month of the release of the surgeon general's report, cigarette sales had dropped by 20 percent. Some states reported declines of more than 30 percent.

But then something unexpected happened. Three months after the release of the surgeon general's report, the tobacco companies were breathing much easier—cigarette sales had in fact returned to their pre-report levels. Regardless of the health risks, it seems, the majority of smokers found the addictive powers of nicotine too great to shake.

NICOTINE ADDICTION

Nicotine is a key component of tobacco, occurring naturally in the chemical makeup of the plant. The first scientific evidence of nicotine's addictive qualities was reported in 1945 in an experiment at the Medical College of Virginia. To conduct the experiment, researchers obtained a strain of tobacco that was specifically bred with low levels of nicotine. They took half their low-nicotine tobacco supply and had cigarettes produced from the batch. For the other half of the batch, the researchers artificially added nicotine, then had that tobacco rolled into cigarettes. Then they recruited 24 smokers and gave them the low-nicotine cigarettes. After a time, the researchers switched the smokers to the high-nicotine cigarettes. The participants never were told which cigarettes they were smoking.

While smoking the low-nicotine cigarettes, most of the smokers exhibited symptoms of what is known today as "nicotine withdrawal." As recounted in Edward M. Brecher's *Licit and Illicit Drugs*, the smokers complained to the researchers about the taste, quality, and "a vague lack in the satisfaction" with their low-nicotine cigarettes. What's more, many participants "definitely missed the nicotine and continued to do so throughout the period (approximately one month). The symptoms experienced . . . for the most part took the form of varying degrees of heightened irritableness, decreased ability to concentrate on mental tasks, a feeling of inner hunger and emptiness . . . in short, virtually the same symptoms experienced by many individuals on stopping smoking."

The smokers themselves couldn't have been less surprised about the experiment's findings. Virtually every heavy smoker who has tried to give up cigarettes has found himself or herself enduring a physical and emotional torture—certainly not on the scale of the withdrawal symptoms suffered by a heroin addict, but enough to ruin anyone's day. Dr. Sigmund Freud, the

SMOKELESS TOBACCO

Smokeless tobacco, also known as chewing tobacco and snuff, has been used by Americans for hundreds of years and at one time was much more popular than cigarettes. In fact, when the R.J. Reynolds Tobacco Company was founded in 1875, its main product was chewing tobacco.

Today, smokeless tobacco is far less popular. According to testimony given before a U.S. House committee in 1994 by Joseph Taddeo, the president of U.S. Tobacco Company, which manufactures the brands of chewing tobacco known as Copenhagen and Skoal, sales of smokeless tobacco are a quarter of what they were a century ago.

In 1996 a Gallup poll found that just 2 percent of Americans "regularly" use chewing tobacco, while another 2.6 percent of Americans admit to "occasionally" using the products. Still, some highly visible role models continue to set a bad example for young people. Baseball players, for example, have long been aficionados of chewing tobacco, and it is not unusual to see a big-league pitcher standing on the mound with a cheek full of tobacco, staring down the batter, the front of his uniform stained with brown streaks from spitting out his chaw.

People thinking of trying smokeless tobacco should know about its health risks. According to the American Council on Science and Health, ingredients of smokeless tobacco include some 28 substances known to cause cancer. The council says users of smokeless tobacco are six times more likely than nonusers to develop cancer of the mouth and pharynx (the tube that connects the mouth and nasal passage) and 50 times more likely than nonusers to develop cancer of the gums and cheeks. All those cancers are classified as "oral" cancers. About 30,000 new cases of oral cancer are diagnosed each year, including 8,000 cases that prove to be fatal.

There are other health risks as well. Smokeless tobacco contains nicotine, which makes it addictive. Plus, people who inadvertently swallow the tobacco juice expose their stomachs to nicotine, which could lead to ulcers. And smokeless tobacco is also known to cause bad breath and stain teeth.

father of psychotherapy, fought unsuccessfully against his nicotine addiction for some 40 years, finally losing the battle in 1939 when he died from cancer at the age of 83. The final few years of his life were agonizing, as he suffered through a series of operations that removed cancerous tumors from his mouth and jaw. Near the end of his life, Freud's condition was exacerbated by heart disease. During one of his many attempts to quit smoking, Freud wrote of his withdrawal symptoms:

> Soon after giving up smoking there were tolerable days. . . . Then there came suddenly a severe affection of the heart, worse than I ever had when smoking. . . . And with it an oppression of mood in which images of dying and farewell scenes replaced the more usual fantasies. . . . The organic disturbances have lessened in the last couple of days; the hypo-manic mood continues. . . . It is annoying for a doctor who has to be concerned all day long with neurosis not to know whether he is suffering from a justifiable or hypochondriacal depression.

As for the tobacco companies, they steadfastly denied that cigarettes were addictive. In fact, in the 1950s the industry set up its own laboratory—the Council on Tobacco Research—which churned out report after report contending that there were no adverse health effects associated with cigarette smoking. And the tobacco companies would stick to that story well into the 1990s.

"A NICOTINE DELIVERY BUSINESS"

Even before the ban on televised ads for cigarettes took effect in 1971, cigarette companies were forced to print warning labels, on cigarette packs as well as on their print advertisements, informing people of the findings of the surgeon general's report. Also, cigarette sales to minors were outlawed, and cigarette vending machines were prohibited in places where minors could gain access to them.

States began levying heavy taxes on cigarette sales, finding them to be a sure source of revenue. It seemed that people were willing to spend whatever it took to obtain their cigarettes, even paying taxes that eclipsed the cost of the cigarettes themselves. Indeed, the average price of a pack of cigarettes rose from 62 cents in 1969 to nearly four dollars by 2004. In some states with particularly heavy cigarette taxes, such as Massachusetts,

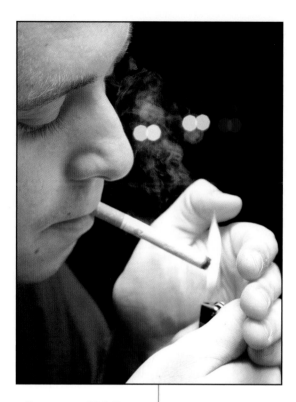

On average, CDC figures show, regular smokers light up about 18 times each day.

smokers today can expect to pay more than six dollars per pack.

None of these measures, however, seemed to curb demand for cigarettes—and public health advocates began to suspect that cigarette manufacturers knew why. In 1994 David Kessler, the commissioner of the U.S. Food and Drug Administration, announced plans to regulate cigarettes as though they were drugs. Kessler suspected that for decades the tobacco companies had been adding nicotine to cigarettes in order to make them even more addictive. By manipulating nicotine levels, he believed, the companies were creating a customer base that was virtually guaranteed to be hooked on their products. Appearing in a PBS *Frontline* program titled "Inside the Tobacco Deal," which first aired in 1998, Kessler said:

I am saying there is evidence that the tobacco companies manipulate nicotine. . . . If you put a filter in front of a cigarette, what's going to get taken out? It's going to filter out the tar. It's also going to filter out the nicotine. Why do people smoke? They smoke for the nicotine. If you take out the tar and you take out the nicotine and you take out too much nicotine people are not going to smoke. So what do you have to do? You have to up the nicotine levels and that, in fact, is what we saw. We saw an industry that was manipulating the level of nicotine in the low delivery cigarettes. And the vast majority of cigarettes sold in this country are low delivery. Light cigarettes are light in what? They're light in tar. They're light in nicotine. We sent light cigarettes to our laboratory and found the light cigarettes have a higher concentration of nicotine than the regular cigarettes. How does that happen? That can't happen without manipulation and control of nicotine.

The tobacco companies vehemently denied the charge.

In 1994 the U.S. House Energy and Commerce Committee convened a series of hearings to air Kessler's plan to regulate tobacco as a drug. Executives from all the major American tobacco companies testified, and they all insisted that smoking was not hazardous to health. In addition, they all stood by the claim that they did not manipulate the levels of nicotine in their cigarettes. At the time of the hearing, it was estimated that some 50 million Americans smoked cigarettes. James Johnston, chairman and chief executive officer of R.J. Reynolds Tobacco Company, testified:

> We do not manipulate nicotine to addict smokers. We no more manipulate nicotine in cigarettes than coffee manufacturers manipulate caffeine in their products. There is nothing sinister about it. I think the [committee] should also be aware that Dr. Kessler's definition of addiction would classify most coffee, cola and tea drinkers as addicts, caffeine addicts. Many people experience a strong urge for a cup of coffee each morning, and there is a well-documented physical withdrawal syndrome associated with the consumption of coffee and caffeinated soft drinks. . . .
>
> Nicotine plays an essential role in the overall smoking experience. It enhances the taste of the smoke and the way it feels on the smoker's palate, and it contributes to overall smoking enjoyment. During the past several years, there have been a wide variety of attempts to convince the American public that cigarettes are addictive, and some public officials have even gone so far as to put cigarettes in the same class as cocaine and heroin. You don't need to be a trained scientist to see this isn't true. All you need do is ask and honestly answer two simple questions. First, would you rather board a plane with a pilot who just smoked a cigarette or one with a pilot who just had a couple of beers or snorted cocaine or shot heroin or popped some pills?
>
> Second, if cigarettes were addictive, could almost 43 million Americans have quit smoking, almost all of them without any outside help?

Unknown to the tobacco companies, though, information they had been suppressing for years—that their own research showed cigarette smoking was addictive—had been leaked to the press and federal officials. In February 1996 Dr. Jeffrey Wigand, a biochemist and former director of research for the Brown & Williamson tobacco company, appeared on the news program *60 Minutes* and told what he knew about the industry's research into the addictive qualities of nicotine. What's more, Wigand said that Brown & Williamson manipulated the levels of nicotine in the company's cigarettes—clearly to hook smokers and make them customers for life. Wigand said he had been assigned by Brown & Williamson to develop a cigarette that would not cause cancer or other ill effects. "People will continue to smoke no matter what, no matter what kind of regulations," Wigand said. "If you can provide for those who are smoking, who need to smoke, something that produces less risk for them, I thought I was going to make a difference."

But, as Wigand related, the company soon abandoned the project to find a safer cigarette. By then, many of the nation's tobacco companies were facing lawsuits filed by smokers, contending that cigarettes caused their debilitating diseases and that they couldn't give up smoking because they were hooked by the nicotine content of the cigarettes. In the view of Brown & Williamson executives, Wigand told *60 Minutes*, actively seeking to manufacture a "less hazardous or safer" cigarette would be tantamount to admitting that the company knew its products were dangerous, which would provide ammunition for the lawsuits.

Wigand said he decided to go public with his accusations because of the testimony the tobacco company executives delivered at the 1994 congressional hearing. He said, "Part of the reason I'm here is I felt that their representation clearly, at least within Brown & Williamson's representation, clearly misstated what they commonly knew as language within the company. That we're a nicotine delivery business."

SUPPLY AND DEMAND

In the meantime, the tobacco companies were facing charges in court. In 1994 Michael Moore, the attorney general of Mississippi, filed a lawsuit against cigarette manufacturers, alleging that their products placed a severe financial burden on the government of Mississippi, which had to provide medical treatment and various social services to people who were suffering from cancer and other diseases associated with smoking. On *60 Minutes*, Moore charged, "I'm used to dealing with, with cocaine dealers and crack dealers and I have never seen damage done like the tobacco company has done. There's no comparison. Cocaine kills [10,000 or] 15,000 people a year in this country. Tobacco kills 425,000 people a year."

Other state attorneys general soon filed their own lawsuits. At first, the tobacco companies vigorously opposed the suits, but as evidence started to surface that supported the contentions of Wigand, Kessler, and others, it became clear that the tobacco companies were going to lose in court. Tobacco executives also feared that the threats by Congress and the Food and Drug Administration to regulate tobacco as a drug also could be devastating to their industry. Indeed, in 1997 William Osteen, a U.S. district judge, ruled that the Food and Drug Administration did have the authority to regulate nicotine as a drug. The tobacco industry immediately appealed Osteen's order, and tobacco

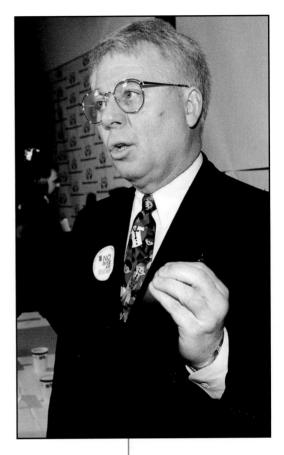

Dr. Jeffrey Wigand, former research director for cigarette manufacturer Brown & Williamson, exposed wrongdoing in the tobacco industry. In 1996 Wigand revealed that, not only had the tobacco industry long been aware of nicotine's addictive qualities, it had manipulated nicotine levels in cigarettes in order to keep users addicted.

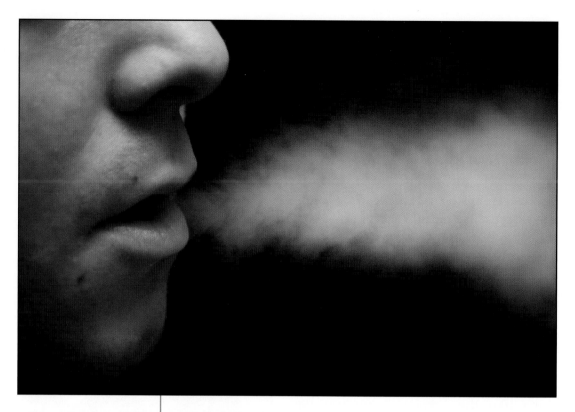

Tobacco smoke contains some 4,000 different chemical compounds, more than 40 of which are known to cause cancer in humans.

executives clearly were concerned about the ramifications of the ruling if the appellate courts upheld it. What would happen if nicotine were treated as a drug? Would a smoker need a prescription from a doctor to obtain a pack of cigarettes? What doctor in America would write a prescription for cigarettes?

With the threat of federal regulation hanging over their heads, and with legal action initiated against them by virtually every state attorney general, the nation's tobacco companies finally caved in. On June 20, 1997, the tobacco companies announced a settlement to the attorneys general suits, by which the companies agreed to pay an enormous $368.5 billion in damages to the states to finance anti-smoking programs and to compensate the states for the costs of caring for terminally ill cancer patients and others suffering from the ill effects of smoking.

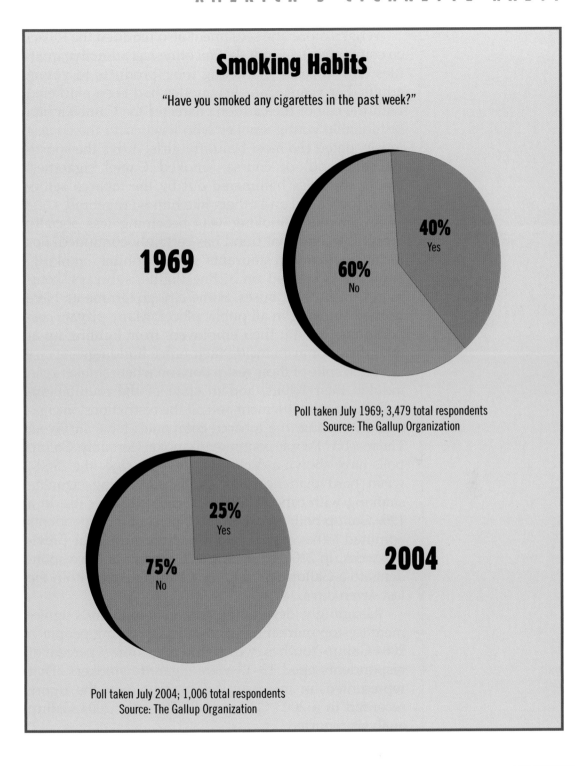

Smoking Habits

"Have you smoked any cigarettes in the past week?"

1969

40%
Yes

60%
No

Poll taken July 1969; 3,479 total respondents
Source: The Gallup Organization

25%
Yes

75%
No

2004

Poll taken July 2004; 1,006 total respondents
Source: The Gallup Organization

What's more, the settlement also required the tobacco companies to admit that nicotine has addictive qualities and to cease marketing their products to young adults. For years, Camel cigarettes had been marketed with the use of the cartoon character Joe Camel, a hip, fashionable young smoker who listened to the coolest music, dated the most beautiful girls, drove the sportiest cars, and, of course, smoked Camel cigarettes. Under the rules hammered out by the tobacco settlement, Joe Camel and others like him were retired.

Meanwhile, smoking was becoming less socially acceptable, and that trend has certainly continued. For instance, many restaurants now prohibit smoking. Smoking is banned on airline flights, subways, commuter trains, and buses. Some city governments have banned smoking in all public places. Many private corporations prohibit their employees from lighting up at their desks or even inside their office buildings.

Yet in spite of these restrictions on where smokers can indulge their habits, and in spite of the multibillion-dollar tobacco settlement and all the restrictions on cigarette marketing, the tobacco companies have survived. The reason? People continue to smoke. Certainly, Gallup polls have shown a decline in smoking since the 1960s, when hard evidence was published linking cigarette smoking with cancer, heart disease, and other ills. In a 1969 Gallup poll, for example, 40 percent of respondents admitted to having smoked cigarettes during the previous week. In 2004, by contrast, 25 percent of the respondents to a Gallup poll said they had smoked within the last seven days.

Alarmingly, despite the tobacco's industry's agreement to stop marketing its products to young people, a 2004 Gallup Youth Survey found that some 9 percent of respondents aged 13–17 were cigarette smokers. That represented an increase of 1 percent over the figure recorded in a 2003 Gallup poll. The May 2004 Gallup analysis reported:

The ALA [American Lung Association] recommends a variety of policies and practices to prevent young people from smoking, including school anti-smoking education, restrictions on advertisements, a ban on smoking on school grounds, enforcing bans on selling tobacco products to those under 18, and providing cessation programs at school, among other things. But perhaps the best way to prevent young people from lighting up is also the simplest—setting a good example. Research shows that kids who live in households in which the adults do not smoke are among those least likely to ever take up the habit in the first place.

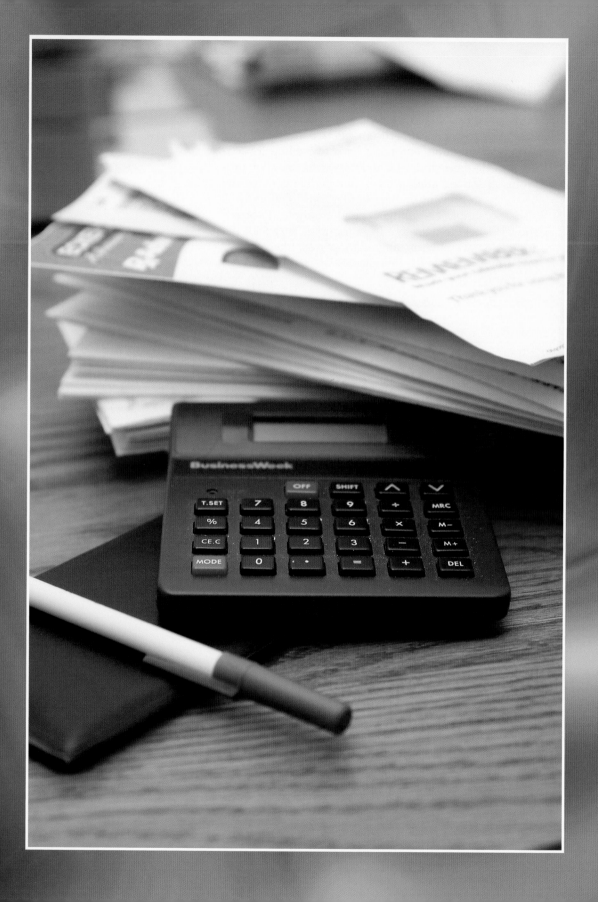

5

THE SPIRALING COST OF HEALTH CARE

In the fall of 1991, a little-known candidate for public office was about to shake the foundations of every hospital, doctor's office, pharmacy, drug manufacturer, and health insurance company in the United States. In fact, the bedrock of America's extremely successful system of delivering health care to its citizens is still shaking, and it doesn't appear the tremors are going to end anytime soon.

The candidate was Harris Wofford, a Democrat who had been appointed to fill a vacant U.S. Senate seat in Pennsylvania after the incumbent, Republican H. John Heinz III, died in an airplane accident. At first, Wofford said he would serve only until a special election could be held to fill the seat, but then he changed his mind and decided to run in the special election. His opponent was Republican Richard Thornburgh, the former two-term governor of Pennsylvania who stepped down as President George H. W. Bush's attorney general to seek the Senate seat.

Most political insiders conceded the seat to Thornburgh. The popular former governor held

(Opposite) Per capita spending on health care is higher in the United States than in any other country. In 2005, according to U.S. government statistics, total health care spending reached $6,423 per person. And, driven by rising costs for medical services and America's aging population, that figure is likely to continue increasing.

a 47-point lead over Wofford in the polls as the race headed into the fall. But Wofford's strategists proved adept at polling and gauging public opinion, and as they floated issues before the electorate that summer they discovered that voters in Pennsylvania were frustrated—in alarmingly high numbers—by one issue in particular: the ever-increasing cost of health care. As a result of the findings, Wofford started airing television commercials in the fall that called for Congress to rein in the high cost of health care. One such commercial featured the candidate standing in front of a busy nurses' station in a hospital, pointing out that while he favored affordable health care, his opponent did not. "The Constitution says that if you are charged with a crime, you have a right to a lawyer," Wofford insisted, according to a *Time* magazine article by Michael Kramer. "But it's even more fundamental that if you're sick, you should have the right to a doctor."

Wofford made affordable health care his issue, and the voters responded. He upset Thornburgh on Election Day—sending a clear message to leaders in Washington that voters were angry and frustrated about the high cost of health care. Although Wofford has since slipped back into obscurity (he lost his next election), the issue of affordable health care remains very much on the national agenda.

The fact is, though, that while health care has remained in the national spotlight, America's political leaders have been able to accomplish very little to make it affordable and available to everyone. As a result, there are millions of Americans who can't afford to go to the doctor. According to the Washington-based National Coalition on Health Care, in 2004 some 45 million Americans—16 percent of the population of the United States—were uninsured.

What is the current system like? In a word, expensive. A routine doctor's office visit, for example, might cost $80 to $100. A visit to a specialist could cost more.

Hospitalization runs into the hundreds or thousands of dollars per day, depending on the type of care provided. High-tech tools such as magnetic resonance imaging (MRI) and computed tomography (CT) scans help physicians see inside the bodies of patients and diagnose problems. Again, however, the cost of an MRI or CT scan can easily exceed $1,000. Even drugs can be expensive; some prescription medications cost hundreds or thousands of dollars per month.

Who pays such costs? For people with health insurance, most medical expenses are paid by a health insurance company. Whenever the individual accesses the health care system—say, to visit a physician or get a prescription filled—he or she is typically required to pay only a modest sum (perhaps $10 or $20) called a co-payment. The doctor, pharmacy, or other service provider will be reimbursed later by the health insurer for the balance of the cost.

But who pays for health insurance? In most cases, health insurance is included in the benefits an employer makes available to employees. Typically, employees contribute to the cost of their insurance, paying a quarter or more of the cost through payroll deductions, but the employer pays most of the cost, and since the employer is likely to be insuring dozens, hundreds, or even thousands of employees, chances are the employer can negotiate lower prices for insurance than could employees if they bought health insurance on their own.

That's how the system is supposed to work, but that's not how things always have worked over the years. The system has a lot of holes in it. For example, because of the spiraling cost of insurance, many smaller companies that are unable to negotiate low rates with insurers have dropped health insurance as a benefit. Similarly, many self-employed people can't afford to buy insurance for themselves and their families. Likewise, those who are unemployed largely are left out of the system.

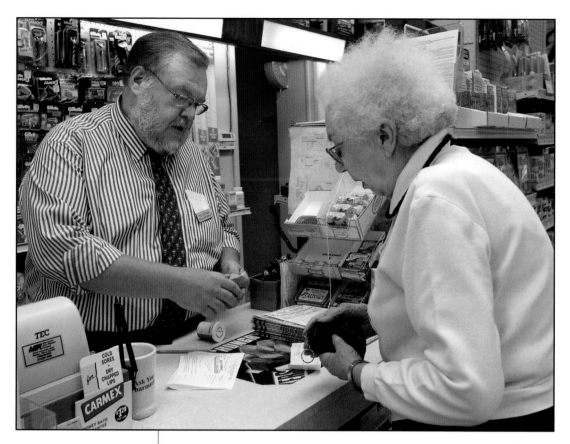

A senior citizen buys her prescription medications at a pharmacy in Chicago. The high cost of prescription drugs has been a major concern for older Americans, many of whom live on fixed incomes and require multiple medications.

Even employees fortunate enough to have health insurance plans have seen their share of the cost rising year after year, taking bigger and bigger bites out of their paychecks. "Basically it's because cost increases for health care outpace family incomes by a factor of two or three," explained William Galston, a University of Maryland political analyst. "The anxiety is increased because more and more employers are requiring more and more employees to pay a higher share of health care costs. What's worse, many people find themselves locked into jobs they don't like simply because they're afraid of losing their existing health plans if they change employment."

There are other deficiencies in the system as well. For example, older Americans who need round-the-clock custodial care often see their life's savings evaporate as they struggle to pay the $50,000 or more per year that it costs them to live in a nursing home. The uninsured—who tend not to have regular doctors—often end up in hospital emergency departments, where care is extremely expensive. Many have routine ailments that could easily be addressed with a much less costly visit to a doctor's office. Others have developed acute or serious conditions that could have been avoided had they obtained routine care earlier. Regardless, hospitals treat these patients, and because they frequently cannot pay for the care provided, hospital costs tend to get passed on to patients who can pay. All of this has helped contribute to a health care delivery system that, in the view of many observers, is badly in need of reform.

SOCIALIZED MEDICINE

Over the years, Gallup polls consistently have shown that Americans believe the government has a responsibility to ensure that health care is affordable. As far back as May 1938, a Gallup poll posed this question: "Do you think the government should be responsible for providing medical care for people who are unable to pay for it?" More than 78 percent of the respondents said yes, and 55 percent were willing to pay higher taxes for that purpose; just 18 percent said no.

Following World War II, President Harry S. Truman proposed a national health insurance plan that would ensure Americans access to doctors, hospitals, and drugs. His plan was opposed immediately and angrily by the nation's physicians, who worried that if the government took over the administration of health care, it would set prices that doctors could charge for their services. The American Medical Association became the main lobbying group for the doctors, pressing members of Congress to oppose Truman's plan, which it labeled "socialized medicine." The AMA sponsored an advertising and publicity campaign designed to "keep public opinion hostile to national health insurance," according to an article in the *Journal of Health and Social Behavior*.

By referring to Truman's plan as "socialized medicine," the AMA and other opponents—including insurance companies, drug manufacturers, and business groups, such as chambers of commerce—sought to play on the public's fears of communism. This was the late 1940s—the dawn of the Cold War, an era when Americans feared Communist infiltration of their society. Even though Americans wanted the government to provide health care for people who could not afford it, a Gallup poll reported in 1949 that 42 percent of Americans disapproved of "socialized medicine," while just 38 percent favored it.

Shortly before the congressional elections of 1950, opponents of Truman's plan also organized campaigns against members of Congress who supported national health insurance. One candidate who felt their wrath was Senator Claude Pepper of Florida, an architect of the Truman plan. A doctor who opposed Pepper circulated a fund-raising letter to his fellow physicians stating, "We physicians in Florida have a terrific fight on our hands to defeat Senator Claude Pepper, the outstanding advocate of 'socialized medicine' and the 'welfare state' in America. In eliminating Pepper from Congress, the first great battle against Socialism in America will have been won."

Doctors contributed substantial sums of money to the campaign against Pepper and even paid for newspaper advertisements showing a photo of the senator standing alongside Paul Robeson, an African American actor, singer, and avowed member of the Communist Party. Pepper as well as five other members of Congress who supported Truman's plan were defeated at the polls that year. Others in Congress got the message, and from then on the idea of national health insurance was received

Government-Sponsored Health Care

"Would you be willing to pay higher taxes so that the government can provide medical care for people who are unable to pay for it?"

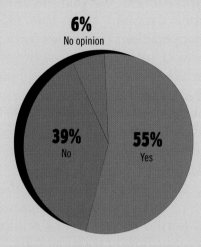

Poll taken May 1938; 3,051 total respondents
Source: The Gallup Organization

Socialized Health Care

"Would you approve or disapprove of socialized medicine in this country?"

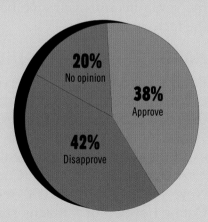

Poll taken February 1949; 2,493 total respondents
Source: The Gallup Organization

coolly on Capitol Hill. Truman left office following the 1952 election, and his successor, President Dwight D. Eisenhower, opposed national health insurance.

Throughout the fight for national health insurance, supporters of the plan included leaders of the nation's labor unions. After the 1950 election, the unions dropped their campaign for a national health plan and instead adopted the tactic of pressing employers to include health insurance benefits in their contracts. That tactic was largely successful. Big companies were much more willing to provide health insurance on their own because they felt they could watch costs more closely than if the government administered a national plan.

Between 1946 and 1957, the number of union workers covered by health insurance plans rose from just 1 million to more than 12 million. Since most plans also covered family members, by 1957 it was believed that some 20 million people were covered by health insurance plans that were negotiated into union contracts. Meanwhile, the so-called white-collar workers who were not members of unions also found themselves beneficiaries of company health plans; they were given the same health insurance benefits as the laborers on the factory floors.

MANDATE FOR SWEEPING CHANGE

But not everybody was covered. People living in poverty had little access to health care. Retired people found themselves without health insurance as well.

By the early 1960s senior citizens were starting to exert themselves as a political force in America. At the 1964 Democratic National Convention in Atlantic City, New Jersey, some 14,000 members of the National Council of Senior Citizens staged a demonstration on the city's boardwalk in front of Convention Hall. Their demands were clear: a national health insurance program designed specifically for them. They found a willing president in Lyndon B. Johnson, who had taken office the year before, following the assassination of President John F. Kennedy. In the 1964 election, Johnson, running against conservative Republican Barry Goldwater, won in a landslide.

Johnson regarded his victory as a mandate to bring sweeping change to American society. He proposed—and easily pushed through Congress—major components of a domestic reform agenda he called the "Great Society." The Great Society programs were designed to lift people out of poverty, end discrimination against minorities, and improve the educational opportunities available to young people. Two of the programs were Medicare and Medicaid. Both would go a long way toward providing medical care to people who, through dire economic circumstances, had been left out of the health care system.

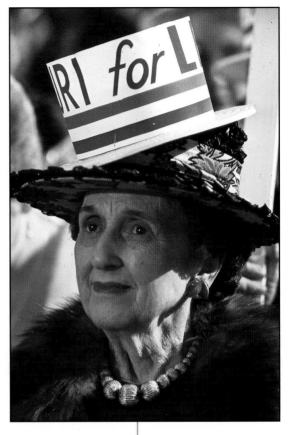

A delegate to the 1964 Democratic National Convention in Atlantic City, New Jersey, shows her support for President Lyndon B. Johnson. Senior citizens had a particularly visible presence at that convention, and upon winning the presidential election Johnson spearheaded the push for a program that has benefited countless elderly Americans: Medicare.

Medicare was designed for elderly people who could not afford their own health care. It was financed through payroll taxes paid by working Americans. Medicare provides hospital care for elderly people, although it covers other services as well. Medicaid covers health care for people of all ages considered too poor to pay their own medical bills. The federal government subsidizes the cost, but state governments also are expected to contribute to Medicaid.

Medicare and Medicaid were comprehensive programs, serving millions of people who had been unable to afford medical care. But costs soon got out of hand. With the government paying the bills, doctors and hospitals suddenly raised their rates. In 1965, the first year Medicare was in effect, the daily cost of hospitalization rose 16 percent. Doctors also raised their prices, by an average of 25 percent. Of course, with medical costs starting to skyrocket, the cost of private health insurance quickly shot up as well. When union leaders went to the bargaining tables, they found corporations demanding that health benefits be scaled back or union members be made to pay greater shares of the insurance.

Once again, the government looked for a way to rein in costs. In 1971 Senator Edward Kennedy of Massachusetts introduced a national plan he called "Health Security," which would place the government in charge of all health care costs. Once again, doctors, hospitals, and others in the business of delivering health care vehemently opposed government control. Over the next three years, Health Security would bounce around Congress, where medical industry lobbyists convinced sympathetic members to water down the legislation.

Meanwhile, the country was mired first in the Vietnam War and then in the Watergate scandal. Affordable health care seemed low on most people's priority lists. Even so, after the Watergate scandal forced the resignation of President Richard M. Nixon in 1974, his successor, President Gerald R. Ford, called on Congress to adopt a national health plan. Ford, a Republican, had no mandate from the voters — he had, essentially, been appointed president — and he certainly had little influence in the Democrat-controlled Congress. He left office in 1977 without ever getting the chance to sign a national health care bill into law. Once again, a national health insurance plan was allowed to die on the vine.

Over the next 15 years, the costs of health care continued to escalate, and more and more people found themselves without coverage. But by 1991, lawmakers were not facing the same issues they had faced in the early 1960s. In the 1960s, they had to find a way to deliver health care to poor and elderly Americans. They responded with Medicare and Medicaid. But by the 1990s, the costs of those two programs were spiraling out of control. In 1965, the first year of Medicare, the program had cost $5 billion. In 1991 it cost $110 billion.

Medicaid costs also had skyrocketed, to a reported $158 billion in 1991. And Medicaid now was covering people it never had covered before. Also, because medical science had helped people live longer, costs for nursing-home patients were rising. By 1991 Medicaid was paying for some 250,000 Americans to live in very expensive institutions that provided them with round-the-clock custodial care—at a cost of $34,000 per person per year. Other problems occurred when women (especially poor, inner-city women) became addicted to crack cocaine. Many of them delivered babies also addicted to crack, and Medicaid financed the care for some 158,000 so-called crack babies a year—at a cost of $1.8 billion. Additionally, the cost of caring for an AIDS patient was so steep that most patients ran through their personal savings in no time, which required Medicaid to step in. By 1991 Medicaid was financing the care for 35,000 AIDS patients.

There were other problems as well. By the early 1990s, juries were routinely awarding plaintiffs large settlements in malpractice lawsuits brought against doctors—in many cases, doctors and insurance companies charged, when the medical care provided had not been substandard. "Medical care is not always successful," fumed Edmund Kelly, the president of the Aetna-U.S. Healthcare insurance company, "but that doesn't mean the doctor should have to pay huge awards for pain and suffering." Actually, doctors who were sued did not themselves pay malpractice awards—the insurance companies who wrote the doctors' malpractice policies did. And as damage awards increased, the insurers hiked the premiums they charged doctors for malpractice coverage. Naturally, the doctors sought to pass at least part of the additional costs on to their patients. Meanwhile, many doctors started practicing what's known as "defensive medicine"—for example, by ordering unnecessary (and expensive) tests—to protect themselves from potential malpractice lawsuits. By the early 1990s, it was estimated that defensive medicine was costing between $21 billion and $132 billion a year.

While the government made sure that the poorest citizens continued to receive health care, by 1991 many middle-class Americans were beginning to find themselves outside the system. With costs escalating, small employers started dropping their employees' health insurance plans—a bitter pill for many workers to swallow. And so when Pennsylvania senator Harris Wofford's political advisers started polling the electorate in the summer of 1991, they discovered that one of every nine Americans was without health insurance, and the vast majority of people still lucky enough to be insured thought that health care was excessively expensive. James Carville, one of Wofford's political strategists, wrote in his book *All's Fair*:

> Health care went to the core of the matter. People were having a hard time taking care of themselves, and the government wasn't doing anything about it. The more we talked about it, the more people responded. It was like, "Finally, somebody in a campaign is talking about something that matters to me." This was not a right-wing flag factory display of empty patriotism—or, on the left, a tangential issue like gays in the military. This was something that was relevant to people's daily lives and you just had a sense that they were excited that somebody was talking about it.

HARRY AND LOUISE

Pennsylvanians weren't the only voters worried about affordable health care; in early 1992, a Gallup poll showed that 80 percent of American voters believed affordable health care should be a very important issue in the coming presidential campaign. As the 1992 race started taking shape, the governor of Arkansas, Bill Clinton, emerged as a front-runner. Clinton not only adopted Wofford's message but also hired the team of political consultants who engineered the Senate candidate's victory over Thornburgh. By then, all the major candidates were talking about affordable health care.

Clinton won the 1992 election and soon made good on his campaign promise to address America's national health care mess. He appointed his wife, Hillary Rodham Clinton, to head the National Task Force on Health Care Reform. The first lady's task force worked on the issue for nearly a year, releasing the "Health Security Plan," which quickly won the president's endorsement, in the fall of 1993. It was an extremely complicated plan that would require government oversight of the health care industry. The plan was designed to be "universal," meaning it would guarantee access to health care for all Americans.

Under the Clinton plan, states would have the authority to set up regional alliances, whose size would enable them to negotiate favorable rates with health insurance providers. Small businesses that otherwise might be priced out of the health insurance market could get affordable coverage for their employees under the umbrella of the regional alliances. Other consumers could also enroll through the alliances to obtain health insurance for themselves and their families. To keep coverage affordable, the government would set rates based on the ability of consumers to pay and would provide subsidies to the states. To help pay the cost of health insurance, the task force recommended a tax on cigarettes of 75 cents per pack.

Intense opposition to the Clinton health care plan surfaced immediately. Doctors, insurance companies, drug companies, hospitals, and others in the business of providing health care attacked the plan for the same reasons they had been attacking proposed national health plans since the Truman years: they insisted that once the government got involved, it would remove the delivery of health care from the free market, thus limiting the fees doctors and hospitals could charge, the premiums insurance companies could collect, and the prices pharmaceutical companies could command for prescription drugs. A fierce political fight broke out on Capitol Hill and across the country over the fate of the Clinton health plan.

In Washington, lobbyists for the health care industry worked to convince members of Congress to vote against the Clinton plan. Meanwhile, ordinary Americans watched a battle for their hearts and minds unfold, as an insurance industry group, the Coalition for Health Insurance Choices, sponsored a series of television ads featuring a middle-class couple, Harry and Louise, fretting over how the federal government wanted to create a huge bureaucracy dictating how every American was to receive health care.

In November 1993, shortly after the task force released details of the plan, a Gallup poll showed Americans willing to accept the Clinton plan by a margin of 52-40. In the same poll, 74 percent of respondents said that Congress should adopt the plan, either as it was written by the task force or with changes. Only 20 percent of respondents favored rejection of the Clinton plan.

But after months of exposure to the Harry and Louise commercials, as well as a constant stream of criticism from conservative commentators, spokespeople for the health care industry, and other sources, the public was far less willing to accept the Clinton plan. In July 1994 a Gallup poll showed support for the Clinton health plan at just 40 percent, with 55 percent of respondents opposed to the plan.

Clearly, public opinion had been influenced by the health care industry's special-interest groups. In March

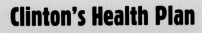

Clinton's Health Plan

"Do you think Congress should pass the Clinton Health Plan as proposed, pass it only after making major changes, or reject it?"

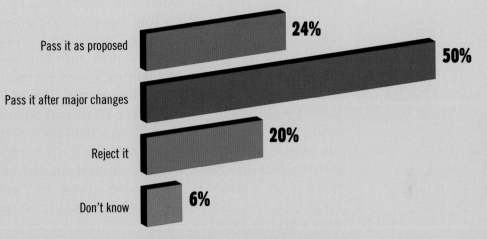

Pass it as proposed **24%**

Pass it after major changes **50%**

Reject it **20%**

Don't know **6%**

Poll taken November 1993; 1,002 total respondents
Source: The Gallup Organization

Approval of Clinton's Plan

"Do you favor or oppose President Clinton's plan to reform health care?"

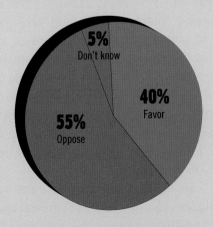

5% Don't know

40% Favor

55% Oppose

Poll taken July 1994; 1,001 total respondents
Source: The Gallup Organization

1994 the *Wall Street Journal* published an article by Hilary Stout titled "Many Don't Realize It's Clinton's Plan They Like." In opinion polls, the article reported, 45 percent of Americans said they were opposed to the Clinton national health care plan, but 76 percent actually endorsed the plan when they were read its major provisions without being told where those provisions came from. Jahan Bashir, a secretary and mother of seven who participated in the poll, said she believed the Clinton plan was too complex and probably too expensive. As reported in the *Journal* article, when Bashir was read the details of the Clinton plan, without being told it was produced by the task force, she said, "It sounds good. Employers may pick up a lot of the burden, but if the employer can't afford it, the government will subsidize. So you're going to have the employer, the government and the insurance companies working together."

Still, President Clinton was unable to muster a majority in Congress to pass his health care plan. A year after the task force proposed the plan, congressional leaders declared it dead. Over the next decade, Congress again would make some efforts to alter the health care system, but the resulting changes fell considerably short of a major overhaul—and, it was generally acknowledged, did little to address the issue of spiraling costs. For example, a law was passed prohibiting insurance companies from rejecting workers because of preexisting conditions (illnesses or handicaps predating acceptance of a new job). And in 2004 Congress passed legislation giving senior citizens a prescription drug benefit under Medicare. That benefit was projected to cost $1.2 trillion between 2006 and 2015.

In 2003 total health care spending in the United States was reported at no less than $1.7 trillion, yet some 45 million Americans remained uninsured. In 2004 the premiums insurance companies charged employers for health benefits rose 11 percent; employers, in turn,

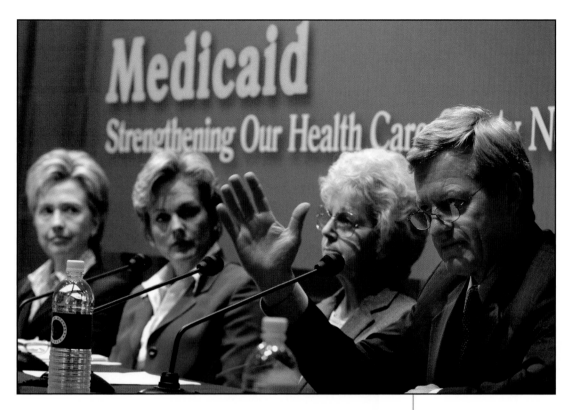

passed virtually the entire cost on to their workers, increasing health insurance payroll deductions by some 10 percent. By 2004 employees were paying an average of 63 percent more for health care benefits than they had paid in 2001. In 2004, according to the National Coalition on Health Care, the average worker with a family of four saw $2,661 withdrawn from his or her annual pay to finance health benefits, while employers contributed an average of $9,950 to pay for each worker's coverage.

AMERICANS NOT SATISFIED

Recent Gallup polls show the continued frustration of Americans who either don't have health insurance or who believe they are paying too much for it. In a November 2005 Gallup poll, 58 percent of respondents said it is the government's responsibility to guarantee

At an April 2005 forum on proposed changes to the Medicaid program are (from left): Senator Hillary Rodham Clinton of New York; Michigan's governor, Jennifer Granholm; Phyllis Craig, a resident of Maine and the sister of an Alzheimer's patient; and Senator Max Baucus of Montana.

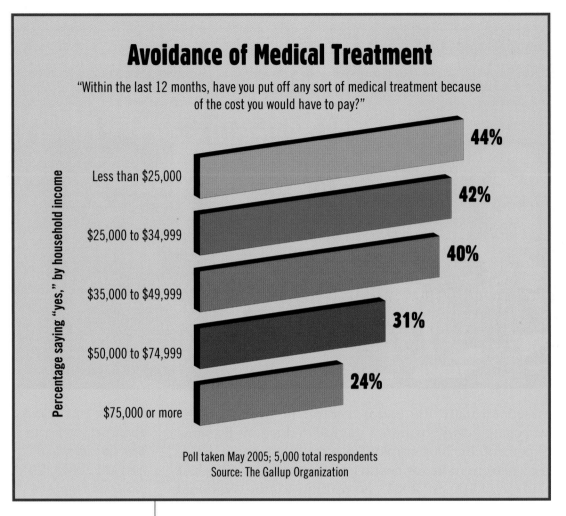

Avoidance of Medical Treatment

"Within the last 12 months, have you put off any sort of medical treatment because of the cost you would have to pay?"

Percentage saying "yes," by household income

Less than $25,000 — 44%

$25,000 to $34,999 — 42%

$35,000 to $49,999 — 40%

$50,000 to $74,999 — 31%

$75,000 or more — 24%

Poll taken May 2005; 5,000 total respondents
Source: The Gallup Organization

affordable health care to citizens, while 34 percent disagreed with that notion. In a separate 2005 poll, people with lower incomes reported far more difficulty obtaining health care. In fact, a large proportion of the respondents—40 percent of those earning $35,000 to $49,999, 42 percent of those earning $25,000 to $34,999, and 44 percent of those earning less than $25,000—said they had to delay medical treatment because of the cost. Dr. Rick Blizzard, a health care consultant for the Gallup Organization, wrote in a Gallup Poll News Service commentary in May 2005:

Reduced access to healthcare services is a financial hardship that threatens Americans' quality of life more directly than any other. Since January [2005], healthcare costs have topped the list when Americans were asked to name the most important financial problem their families face.

Gallup recently conducted a special survey of almost 5,000 members of The Gallup Poll Panel, to gauge their opinions on several healthcare issues. One result in particular jumped out at me: Just 6% reported being satisfied with the total cost of healthcare in the United States. . . . More than 7 in 10 (71%) were dissatisfied— including 46% who said they were "not at all" satisfied. . . .

Americans are highly dissatisfied with the cost of healthcare and this is affecting their behavior when it comes to getting healthcare. As importantly, income has become a serious barrier to accessing needed services. In other words, these data help confirm that the barrier to services is greatest among the populations most likely to need them.

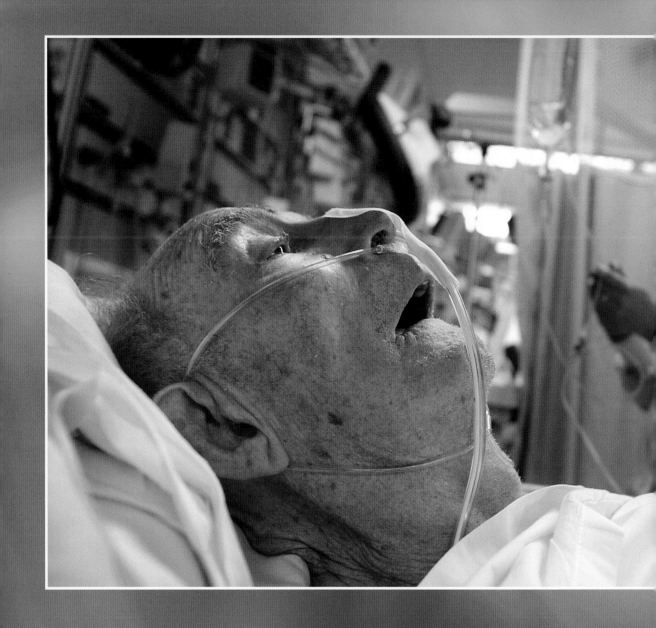

6 THE RIGHT TO DIE

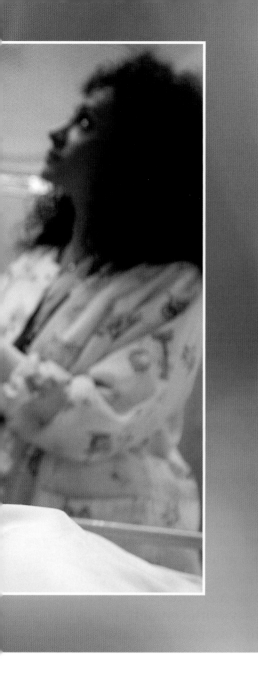

When the Turners of Charlotte, North Carolina, gathered for Mother's Day dinner in 2004, 73-year-old Andrew Turner made a rather startling announcement. "This is my last meal," he told the family, as John Schwartz reported in a *New York Times* story.

Afflicted with colon cancer, Andrew Turner had endured months of pain. As the cancer took its toll, Turner's body wasted away: he dropped from 201 pounds to a mere 130. Finally, Turner advised his family that he no longer wished to live and that he would refuse further cancer treatments. What's more, Turner said he also planned to have his feeding tube removed. He had researched methods of ending his own life and settled on starvation, since very sick people often lose interest in eating altogether. "If you have any comments about that I will listen to them, but this is my decision," he said, according to the *Times*.

Over the next five weeks, Andrew Turner grew weaker while his pain intensified. Doctors prescribed doses of morphine to ease his suffering. Finally, after five weeks, Turner was too weak to rise from bed. As reported in the *Times*, he told his daughter Lise, "I think this is pretty much going to be the weekend that I die."

Andrew Turner lingered for another day. When it became clear that the end was near, his family members gathered around his bed. "We all piled into the bed; we all held on to him and said goodbye," Lise Turner told the *Times*. Lise Turner said she believed her father had made the right decision, and that members of the Turner family were comforted knowing that he had died peacefully. "I think when you've done it right, whatever 'right' means, you feel good," she said.

Nobody knows precisely how many Americans, like Andrew Turner, elect to end their lives in a given year rather than endure painful and debilitating illnesses, but the number is surely in the thousands. While some patients elect to commit suicide in the conventional sense—they may use a gun on themselves or deliberately take a fatal overdose of medication—it has become much more common for patients to elect the course Andrew Turner chose: to stop taking treatment and nourishment. Dr. Ezekiel J. Emanuel, a bioethicist at the National Institutes of Health, noted this trend. During the past 10 to 15 years, Emanuel said, a patient electing to end his own life by dropping a regimen of treatment has gone "from . . . being a contentious issue to . . . being the norm." Gallup polls show that years ago, most Americans opposed the notion of legal suicide for terminally ill patients. In 1947 just 37 percent of Americans favored a law permitting suicide for a terminally ill person, while 52 percent opposed such a law.

Andrew Turner was able to make his own decision about when to terminate his life. Although cancer had devastated his body, his mind was still sharp and he was able to give the issue considerable thought. But what happens when illness or accident leaves a patient unable to make his or her own decisions—for example, in the case of a person suffering from Alzheimer's disease?

Because none of us can say with certainty that we will never become mentally incapacitated, attorneys advise all adults to make appropriate plans, even if they are currently in good health. Typically, people draw up "living wills" or "advance directives," legal documents that give instructions to their family members as well as to physicians on the circumstances under which they want to be kept alive in the event they become incapacitated and unable to make decisions. In living wills, many people advise their family members that they do not want to be kept alive by artificial means—either through mechanical breathing devices or feeding tubes inserted down their throats. By making that provision in their living wills, they assert their "right to die."

A GOOD DEATH

The issue of a patient's right to die has confronted family members, the courts, and lawmakers for years. In 1976 the case of Karen Ann Quinlan brought the issue into the national spotlight.

The previous year, Quinlan, then 21 years old, had suffered respiratory failure and irreversible brain damage after ingesting tranquilizers and alcohol at a party. After the unconscious young woman was taken to the hospital, doctors put her on a respirator to regulate her breathing. As the days and weeks passed, however, it became apparent that the comatose Quinlan would never regain consciousness; she was, in fact, declared "brain dead." With no hope that their daughter would ever recover, Karen Ann Quinlan's parents asked the hospital to remove her from the respirator so that she might "die with dignity." When the hospital refused, the Quinlans sued, contending that the hospital's decision violated their right to privacy. In a decision handed down in March 1976, a year after Karen Quinlan had slipped into a coma, the New Jersey Supreme Court agreed. The court ordered the hospital to remove Quinlan's respirator. (In a turn of events that surprised medical experts, however, Karen Ann Quinlan lived for another nine years.)

In 1990 the United States Supreme Court backed the right to die when it ruled in a Missouri case that a patient has the right to turn down life-sustaining treatment. In the case of Nancy Cruzan, who suffered severe brain damage in a car accident, the Court found that there had been evidence Cruzan did not wish to be kept alive by artificial means, and her family was permitted to remove her feeding tube.

Meanwhile, in Michigan, an eccentric physician named Jack Kevorkian raised the notion of "physician-assisted suicide." Kevorkian realized that many seriously or terminally ill people could use the help of a doctor to end their lives. Although he had been a physician since 1952, Kevorkian had hardly carved out a successful practice. In fact, specializing in pathology—the study of the effects of disease on the body—Kevorkian had developed some rather outlandish notions. For example, in 1961 he suggested that it might be practical to perform blood transfusions from cadavers to live patients.

In the late 1970s, Kevorkian gave up pathology and sank his life savings into the production of a movie, which flopped. He also tried his hand at inventing, developing disposable sun visors as well as a bicycle that sailed through the water on paddle wheels. Eventually, Kevorkian started writing articles for medical journals, arguing in favor of euthanasia. (The word is drawn from the Greek term for "a good death.") One article, titled "The Last Fearsome Taboo: Medical Aspects of Planned Death," envisioned a series of suicide clinics in operation throughout the United States. In 1989, using scrap parts he scrounged from garage sales and hardware stores, Kevorkian fashioned a "suicide machine" on the kitchen table of his apartment in Royal Oak, Michigan.

On June 4, 1990, Janet Adkins, a 54-year-old resident of Portland, Oregon, met Kevorkian in a park near Holly, Michigan. Adkins suffered from the early stages of Alzheimer's disease. There is no cure for Alzheimer's, and it is likely that Adkins would have spent many years slowly losing her memory and eventually would have required round-the-clock custodial care before the disease finally claimed her life.

Reclining on a pallet in the back of Kevorkian's van, Adkins had her arm connected to Kevorkian's suicide machine by a rubber hose. "Have a nice trip," Kevorkian told her, according to a *Vanity Fair* article by

Jack Lessenberry. Adkins then flipped the switch on the machine, and a lethal dose of potassium chloride flowed into her bloodstream. Her death was quick and painless. Her last words to Kevorkian, Lessenberry reported, were "Thank you, thank you." A year later, Kevorkian provided his suicide machine to help end the lives of two other terminally ill patients, Sherry Miller and Marjorie Wantz. In all three cases, he videotaped his sessions with the patients. The camera showed the patients giving Kevorkian heartfelt thanks for helping them end their suffering.

For his involvement in the suicides, Kevorkian was charged with three counts of murder, but in all three cases the charges were thrown out. The judges ruled that there were no laws against assisting suicide in Michigan. In 1992 Kevorkian helped three other terminally ill patients end their lives. Late that year, the

Dr. Jack Kevorkian discusses euthanasia on a television talk show, August 1991. Sitting beside Kevorkian is Marjorie Wantz, a terminally ill victim of pelvic disease. Two months after this appearance, Kevorkian helped Wantz commit suicide.

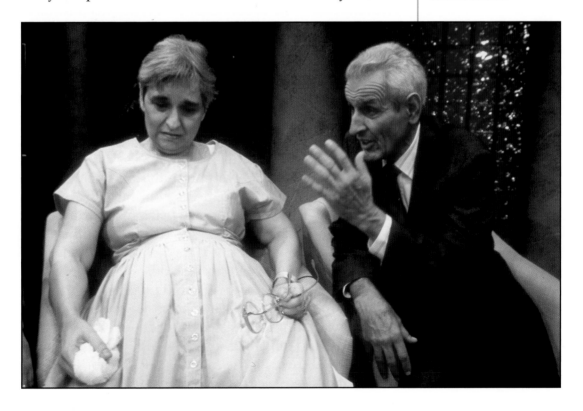

Michigan legislature adopted a law prohibiting assisted suicide, making it a crime punishable by up to four years in prison. The law was scheduled to take effect March 30, 1993. In the eight weeks leading up to the effective date of the law, Kevorkian helped another nine terminally ill patients end their lives.

Shortly after the law took effect, Kevorkian helped end the life of another person. Thomas Hyde, 30 years old, was afflicted with amyotrophic lateral sclerosis (ALS) — which is also known as Lou Gehrig's disease, after the Hall of Fame baseball player who suffered from the fatal ailment. When he was diagnosed with ALS, Hyde, a robust construction worker, was told how the disease would progress: His muscle control would degenerate, and he soon would lose his ability to walk and speak. He would have to be fed through a straw. He would lose control of his bowels. He would be in constant pain from severe cramps. Hyde was informed that many ALS sufferers choke to death on their own saliva. Through it all, though, his mind would remain clear. He would be well aware of his predicament.

As with his other patients, Kevorkian videotaped the final few minutes of Hyde's life. "I want to end this," Hyde says on the tape. "I want to die."

Following Hyde's death, Kevorkian was arrested and charged with violating Michigan's assisted-suicide law. While out on bail awaiting trial, Kevorkian helped two other terminally ill patients commit suicide. One was Dr. Ali Khalili, an Illinois physician suffering from bone cancer. Khalili had access to drugs to end his own life, but in a show of support for Kevorkian, he let the Michigan doctor assist in his suicide.

The videotape made of Hyde before his death moved jurors to acquit Kevorkian. Meanwhile, Michigan's law banning assisted suicide endured many court tests and reversals until, finally, the legislature was forced to rewrite the law. By 1998 Kevorkian had assisted in the suicides of some 100 terminally ill patients. He also had been tried in many deaths and consistently won acquittals; jurors refused to convict him in what they regarded as missions of mercy.

In 1998, though, the television news program *60 Minutes* aired a videotape of the death of Thomas Youck, a 52-year-old sufferer of Lou Gehrig's disease. Unlike the other videotapes, which merely showed Kevorkian providing the suicide machine to the patients, who then flipped the switch themselves, in this instance Kevorkian was seen actually administering the deadly drug to Youck. Kevorkian was charged with murder and with violating the state's assisted-suicide law, and this time he was convicted. In 1999 the doctor was sentenced to a prison term of 10 to 25 years.

RELIGIOUS FAITH

What was the general public's view on assisted suicide and Kevorkian's actions? In 1950, many years before Kevorkian was in the news for aiding in suicides, just 36 percent of respondents told a Gallup poll they supported physician-assisted suicide, while 56 percent opposed it. On the eve of Kevorkian's trial in the death of Thomas Youck, though, public opinion had shifted toward support for physician-assisted suicide. Indeed, in 1999, 52 percent of respondents supported Kevorkian's conduct, while just 43 percent disapproved. Shortly after Kevorkian was convicted, however, a Gallup poll showed a nearly even split in public opinion, with 46 percent of respondents saying the jurors had made the wrong decision, and 44 percent saying the jurors had made the right decision.

Kevorkian's imprisonment did not end the debate. While Michigan's law was undergoing court tests, 43 other states also adopted statutes banning physician-assisted suicide. One state, Virginia, has adopted a measure that permits people who assist in suicide to be sued in civil court. Three states—North Carolina, Utah, and Wyoming—have no laws on the books addressing

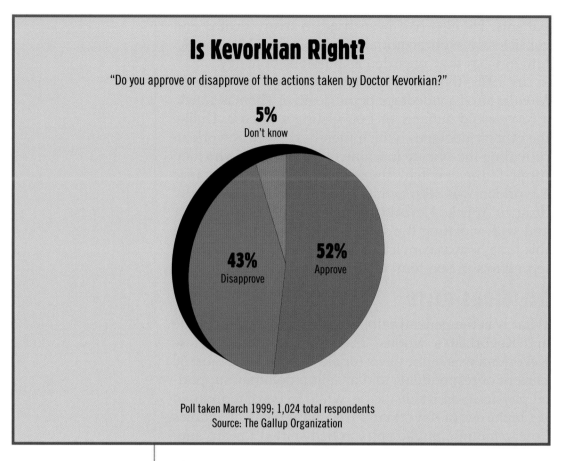

Is Kevorkian Right?

"Do you approve or disapprove of the actions taken by Doctor Kevorkian?"

5%
Don't know

43%
Disapprove

52%
Approve

Poll taken March 1999; 1,024 total respondents
Source: The Gallup Organization

physician-assisted suicide. In Ohio, the state supreme court ruled that physician-assisted suicide is not a crime.

Only Oregon has adopted a law permitting physician-assisted suicide. In referenda held in 1994 and 1997, voters approved of the measure, and by 2005 a total of 208 terminally ill Oregonians had obtained "suicide drugs" from physicians. Under Oregon's law, only mentally competent adults who declare their intentions in writing and are diagnosed as terminally ill may obtain the drugs. The law prohibits doctors from actively participating in a suicide by assisting in "lethal injection, mercy killing or active euthanasia." Oregon's law has been challenged by the U.S. Justice Department, which has argued that the measure violates federal laws prohibiting the distribution of certain drugs or "controlled substances." In early 2005 the U.S. Supreme Court agreed to hear the case, and a decision was expected in 2006.

> Dramatic differences were found according to levels of religiousness or spirituality. According to the 1997 survey, those who most opposed legalizing physician-assisted suicide were people who place the highest importance on their religious faith as an influence in their lives; those who say their life belongs to God or a higher power than to themselves, their families or the community around them; and those who say they are "born-again."
>
> Legalizing physician-assisted suicide was opposed by 68% of those who said that their religious faith is the most important influence in their lives, but by only 11% of those for whom their religious faith is not an important influence in their lives. Similarly, legalizing physician-assisted suicide is opposed by 46% of those who say that their life belongs to God or a higher power but by only 13% of those who say their life belongs to themselves. Fifty percent of those who describe themselves as born-again oppose making physician-assisted [suicide] legal for any reason, compared to 19 percent of those who do not describe themselves that way. . . .
>
> The difference of opinion on physician-assisted suicide between religious and non-religious Americans may lie in the fact that this is part of a larger issue concerning the right to die. Defenders of personal liberty maintain that everyone is morally entitled to end their lives when they see fit. For those people, suicide is morally permissible. While suicide in any form is generally regarded as a sin among Christians and those of many other religions, there is nevertheless a broad range of views among religious Americans.

PERSISTENT VEGETATIVE STATE

Disagreement over the "right to die" would boil over in an acrimonious national debate during the spring of 2005, when the husband of a brain-damaged Florida woman won a court order permitting him to withdraw her feeding tube. The Florida woman, Terri Schiavo, had slipped into what doctors described as a "persistent vegetative state" in 1990, after she suffered a heart attack that denied oxygen to her brain. She was not in a coma and could breathe on her own; nevertheless, she was unresponsive, bedridden, and incapable of swallowing, so she had to be nourished through a feeding tube. Physicians concluded that her condition would never improve. Schiavo's husband, Michael, first asked for her feeding tube to be removed in 1998, but Schiavo's parents, Robert and Mary Schindler, opposed ending her life and insisted that with care their daughter's physical condition could improve.

Terri Schiavo had not prepared a living will. In such cases, the courts usually allow the nearest kin — in this

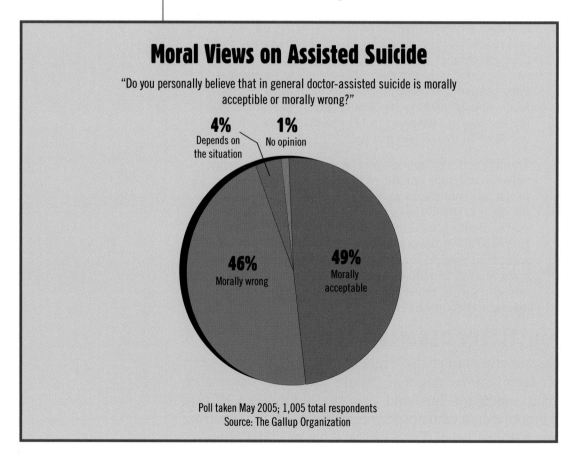

Moral Views on Assisted Suicide

"Do you personally believe that in general doctor-assisted suicide is morally acceptable or morally wrong?"

4%
Depends on
the situation

1%
No opinion

46%
Morally wrong

49%
Morally
acceptable

Poll taken May 2005; 1,005 total respondents
Source: The Gallup Organization

case, her husband—to decide whether to continue artificial life support. Michael Schiavo insisted that before her heart attack, Terri had told him she did not want to be kept alive by artificial means. Initially, the courts ruled in favor of Michael Schiavo, but the Schindlers filed challenges and appeals and the case dragged on for years.

In all the appeals, the courts consistently upheld Michael Schiavo's right to withdraw his wife's feeding tube. By early 2005 all the Schindlers' appeals had been exhausted. In March a judge dismissed the final arguments filed by the Schindlers' attorneys, and on March 18, the feeding tube was removed. At most, doctors gave Terri Schiavo two weeks to live.

By then, however, the Schiavo case had evolved into a national story. Hours after Terri Schiavo's feeding tube was removed, conservative members of Congress took the unusual step of crafting legislation specifically intended to help the Schindlers win a fresh review by the courts. Until then, the state courts in Florida provided most of the rulings in the Schiavo case, but under the emergency legislation passed by Congress and signed by the president, the federal courts would have jurisdiction over the case.

The 11th-hour act of Congress sparked a debate in Washington and across the country. Members of Congress who opposed the law complained that the federal government had inserted itself into what should be a private family matter. House Minority Leader Nancy Pelosi, a member of the Democratic leadership on Capitol Hill, charged: "The actions of the majority in attempting to pass constitutionally dubious legislation are highly irregular and an improper use of legislative authority. Michael Schiavo is faced with a devastating decision, but having been through the proper legal process, the decision for his wife's care belongs to him and to God." Republican Bill Frist, the Senate majority leader, saw the situation differently.

By 2003, when this photo was taken, Terri Schiavo had been in a "persistent vegetative state" for more than a dozen years—the result of oxygen deprivation to her brain following heart failure. In 2005 Schiavo was at the center of a national controversy as her husband, Michael, sought to have her feeding tube removed while her parents, Robert and Mary Schindler, tried to stop him.

"These are extraordinary circumstances," Frist asserted, "that center on the most fundamental of human values and virtues: the sanctity of human life."

Most Americans sided with Michael Schiavo. In a Gallup poll taken as the Florida court ordered the removal of the feeding tube, 56 percent of respondents favored withdrawal of life support for the Florida woman, while just 31 percent argued that the feeding tube should remain in place. What's more, Americans felt that Congress was wrong to enact the emergency legislation. In a poll commissioned by *Time* magazine, an overwhelming majority—75 percent—said the action by Congress and the president to inject themselves into the case was wrong, while just 20 percent agreed with the 11th-hour measure.

"CALM, PEACEFUL AND GENTLE"

A day after Congress passed the legislation transferring the case to the federal courts, Judge James D.

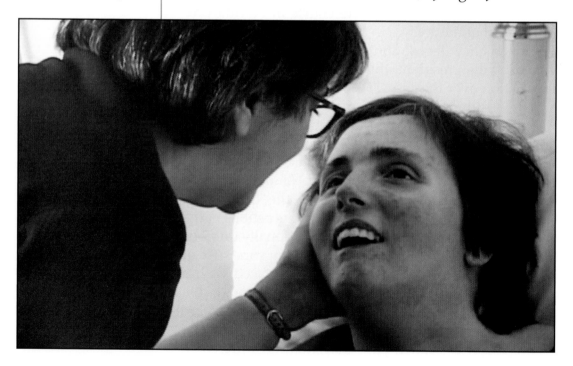

Whittemore held a hearing in which the Schindlers' attorneys argued for the reinsertion of their daughter's feeding tube. A day later, Whittemore issued his ruling. He found that the Schindlers had failed to raise any new issues that would convince him that Terri's husband should be denied the right to have her feeding tube removed. The Schindlers quickly filed appeals, but by the end of the week two federal appellate courts refused to overturn Whittemore's order. Finally, the U.S. Supreme Court refused to hear the case.

On March 31 — 13 days after her feeding tube was removed — Terri Schiavo died. George J. Felos, the attorney who represented Michael Schiavo in most of the court battles, addressed reporters that day. He told them that Michael had been with his wife during the final moments of her life and that as she drew her last breaths, he cradled her in his arms. He described Terri's death as "calm, peaceful and gentle."

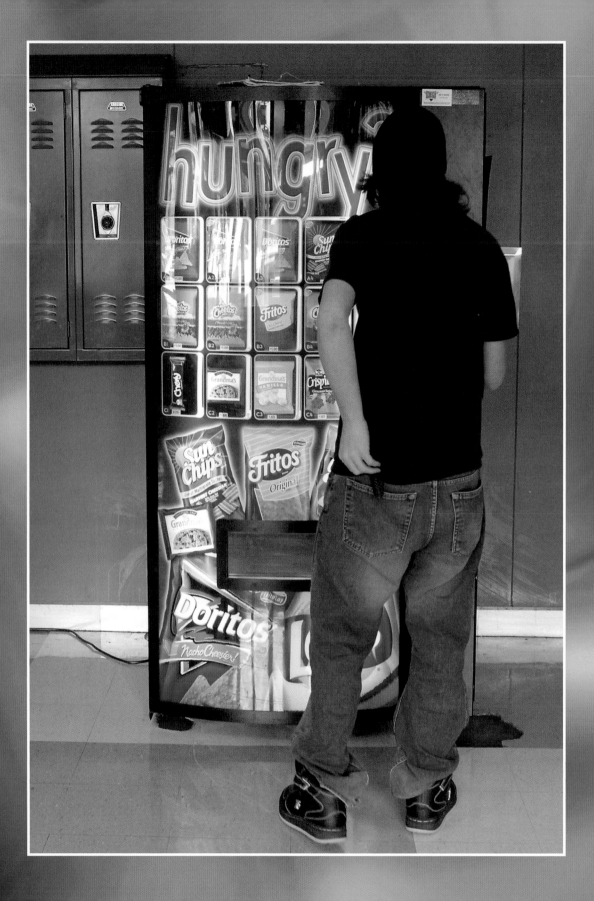

NEW THREATS TO PUBLIC HEALTH

While modern medical science has found ways to extend life, there always will be new threats to health and new challenges for medicine. Overcoming disease, as the conquests of polio and tuberculosis show, often can take decades, and certainly the current fights against AIDS and Alzheimer's disease aren't likely to end soon. Americans may have to wait many years before cures or vaccines become available—if, in fact, they ever are developed at all.

What is most troubling, though, is that Americans often imperil their own health by the lifestyles they choose. The one in four Americans who smoke cigarettes provide perhaps the most obvious example.

Motorcycle owners who insist on riding their bikes without crash helmets provide another example. By 2004 just 19 states required all motorcycle riders to wear helmets, while most other states required some riders—generally those under 18—to wear helmets. In states where helmets are not mandatory, many riders elect not to wear them. And yet, the National

(Opposite) Obesity is an increasingly common problem among young people in the United States. The easy availability of junk food, such as vending machine snacks sold in schools, is but one factor contributing to this trend.

107

Highway Traffic Safety Administration (NHTSA) has concluded that a motorcyclist who does not wear a helmet is 40 percent more likely to suffer a fatal head injury in the event of a crash. Between 1984 and 2002, the NHTSA estimated that the lives of some 14,000 motorcycle riders involved in accidents were saved because they had been wearing their helmets. During that same period, the NHTSA said, 9,500 motorcyclists who died would have survived if they had worn helmets.

While a relatively small segment of the American population rides motorcycles, everybody eats. In recent years, statistics show that many Americans eat too much and are placing themselves at risk due to the health consequences that result from obesity. According to the Centers for Disease Control and Prevention, some 64 percent of Americans over the age of 20 are overweight, and some 30 percent are obese.

The tool by which the CDC determines who may be overweight or obese is body mass index (BMI). This mathematical formula divides weight in kilograms by height in meters squared. Translated into inches and pounds, it means, for example, a six-foot-tall man who weighs 162 pounds has a BMI of 22, which is in the normal range. But a six-foot-tall man who weighs 191 pounds has a BMI of 26, which is in the overweight range. And if a man of the same height weighs 258 pounds, he would have a BMI of 35, which is in the obese range.

Some doctors recommend a less scientific method for determining obesity. They suggest that people look at themselves in the mirror: if they look fat, they probably are fat.

A 2005 study released by Children's Hospital in Boston found that the problem of obesity is growing among young people. The study reported that 16 percent of American children are overweight and another 15 percent risk becoming overweight. Overweight and obese people run the risk of developing diabetes as well as high blood pressure and high cholesterol, which can lead to heart disease. Dr. David S. Ludwig, an author of the Children's Hospital study, warned, "Obesity is such that this generation of children could be the first basically in the history of the United States to live less healthful and shorter lives than their parents. We're in the quiet before the storm. It's like what happens if suddenly a massive number of young children started chain smoking. At first you wouldn't see much public health impact, but years later it would translate into emphysema, heart disease and cancer."

PERCEPTIONS AND REALITY

Most Americans agree with Ludwig's assessment. According to the results of a Gallup Poll Panel released in May 2005, more than half (53 percent) of American adults concede that they are overweight, including 8 percent who regard themselves as "very" overweight. And, judging by statistics from the Centers for Disease Control and Prevention, the situation is actually considerably worse than Americans think—particularly with regard to very overweight individuals. As Gallup health care consultant Dr. Rick Blizzard stated in the poll's commentary, "perceptions are at odds with reality" and "many Americans may be in denial about their weight problems—or at least have a higher threshold for 'overweight' than the clinical CDC definition." Blizzard wrote:

> The specific negative health consequences of being overweight or obese may vary from person to person, and medical community is currently debating the number of deaths that can be attributed to obesity each year. But there is certainly no question that carrying extra weight is not really good for your health.

> Among Americans who rate their personal physical health as either "fair" or "poor," 52% say they are somewhat overweight and 18% say very overweight. Among

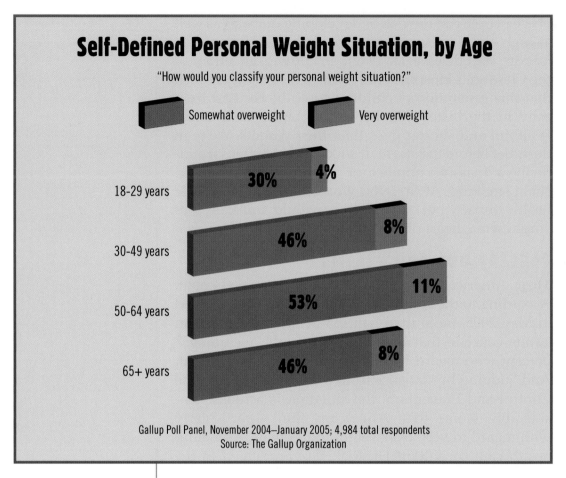

Self-Defined Personal Weight Situation, by Age

"How would you classify your personal weight situation?"

■ Somewhat overweight   ■ Very overweight

18-29 years   30%   4%

30-49 years   46%   8%

50-64 years   53%   11%

65+ years   46%   8%

Gallup Poll Panel, November 2004–January 2005; 4,984 total respondents
Source: The Gallup Organization

those who say they are in "excellent" or "good" physical health, 44% say they are somewhat overweight and 7% say they are very overweight.

Reducing the prevalence of obesity to less than 15% of Americans by 2010 is one of the CDC's main public health objectives. A large majority of Americans would like to work toward achieving that objective—almost 7 in 10 (69%) say they want to lose weight.

How can the health community support and foster this desire to shed unwanted pounds? Medical professionals need to continue to work against the false perception that there is a "quick fix" for obesity—and seek ways to improve Americans' self-discipline regarding the lifestyle changes that are the true long-term solution.

And so, as America moves further into the 21st century, a main challenge for the medical community is not the development of a miracle cure or new drug that would instantly make the pounds melt off the bodies of obese Americans, but to find a way to explain to people that their best hope of living long and healthy lives rests for the most part in the way they choose to live.

antibodies—proteins in the blood that neutralize toxins, thus creating an immunity.

arthritis—a painful inflammation of the joints.

bacteria—one-celled organisms that often carry disease.

bioethicist—a person, often a physician, who studies ethical issues that arise because of advances in medicine, such as whether it is proper for a doctor to assist in a suicide.

bronchitis—an inflammation of the mucous lining of the air passageways leading to the lungs.

cadaver—a dead body.

cholesterol—crystal-like solids found in fats; cholesterol can line the arteries, cutting off blood to the heart and other organs.

emphysema—unnatural elongation of the lungs, resulting in collapse of air passages and obstruction of breathing.

euthanasia—the killing of a person suffering from a painful and incurable disease; also known as mercy killing.

hemophiliac—a person who suffers from excessive bleeding due to a condition that prevents coagulation of the blood.

morphine—a drug derived from opium that is effective in deadening pain.

sputum—saliva mixed with mucus expelled by patients with respiratory ailments.

virus—a microscopic infective agent that is capable of multiplying only in living cells and that causes disease.

Balkin, Karen, ed. *Health Care: Opposing Viewpoints*. Farmington Hills, Mich.: Greenhaven Press, 2003.

Barlett, Donald L., and James B. Steele. *Critical Condition: How Health Care in America Became Big Business—and Bad Medicine*. New York: Doubleday, 2004.

Barry, John M. *The Great Influenza: The Epic Story of the Deadliest Plague in History*. New York: Viking Books, 2004.

Critser, Greg. *Fat Land: How Americans Became the Fattest People in the World*. Boston: Mariner Books, 2004.

Dash, Paul, and Nicole Villemarette-Pittman. *Alzheimer's Disease*. New York: American Academy of Neurology Press, 2005.

Dormandy, Thomas. *The White Death: A History of Tuberculosis*. New York: New York University Press, 2000.

Dworkin, Gerald, and R. G. Frey. *Euthanasia and Physician-Assisted Suicide: For and Against*. New York: Cambridge University Press, 1998.

Gately, Iain. *Tobacco: A Cultural History of How an Exotic Plant Seduced Civilization*. New York: Grove Press, 2003.

Kirby, Michael. *The AIDS Pandemic: Complacency, Injustice, and Unfulfilled Expectations*. Chapel Hill: University of North Carolina Press, 2004.

Oshinsky, David M. *Polio: An American Story*. New York: Oxford University Press-USA, 2005.

Sinclair, Upton. *The Jungle: The Uncensored Original Edition*. Tucson, Ariz.: See Sharp Press, 2003.

http://www.gallup.com

The website of the national polling institute includes polling data and analyses on hundreds of topics.

http://www.ibiblio.org/nhs/NHS-T-o-C.html

The report of the task force headed by Hillary Rodham Clinton to propose an affordable national health insurance plan can be accessed on this site, which is maintained by Ibiblio, a nonprofit group based in Chapel Hill, North Carolina.

http://www.highwaysafety.org

A list of state laws that regulate use of motorcycle helmets can be accessed on this website maintained by the Insurance Institute for Highway Safety.

http://www.jeffreywigand.com

A former tobacco company scientist, Dr. Wigand has become an advocate for a smoke-free society.

http://www.trudeauinstitute.org

The institute, established by Dr. Edward Livingston Trudeau to explore cures for tuberculosis, maintains an extensive archive of articles, tracing the history of the disease as well as the treatment center Dr. Trudeau established in New York's Adirondacks.

Publisher's Note: The websites listed in this book were active at the time of publication. The publisher is not responsible for websites that have changed their address or discontinued operation since the date of publication. The publisher reviews and updates the websites each time the book is reprinted.

BOOKS AND PERIODICALS

Belluck, Pam. "Children's Life Expectancy Being Cut Short by Obesity." *New York Times*, March 17, 2003.

Blizzard, Rick. "Costs Hurt Those Who Need Health Care Most." Gallup Poll News Service, May 3, 2005.

————. "Obesity Epidemic: Are Americans in Denial?" Gallup Poll News Service, May 24, 2005.

Brecher, Edward M. *Licit and Illicit Drugs*. Mount Vernon, N.Y.: Consumers Union, 1972.

Carlson, Darren K. "Americans Call Bioterrorism Most Urgent U.S. Health Problem." Gallup Poll News Service, Nov. 26, 2001.

Castro, Janice. "Condition Critical: Millions of Americans Have No Medical Coverage and Costs Are Out of Control." *Time*, Nov. 25, 1991.

Cowley, Geoffrey. "How to Live to 100." *Newsweek*, June 30, 1997.

Gallup, George. "Many Fear AIDS Epidemic, Expect No Immediate Cure." Gallup Poll, July 7, 1983.

Gallup, George H., Jr. "2 in 3 Would Permit Children to Attend School with AIDS Victim." Gallup Poll, April 17, 1986.

————. "Views on Doctor-Assisted Suicide Follow Religious Lines." Gallup Poll News Service, Sept. 10, 2002.

Grob, Gerald N. *The Deadly Truth: A History of Disease in America*. Cambridge, Mass.: Harvard University Press, 2002.

"The Healing Soil." *Time*, Nov. 7, 1949.

Hill, Miriam. "Drug Seduces Many to Reckless Behavior." *Philadelphia Inquirer*, Feb. 15, 2005.

Hulse, Carl, and David D. Kirkpatrick. "Moving Quickly, Senate Approves Schiavo Measure." *New York Times*, March 21, 2005.

Kramer, Michael. "The Voters' Latest Ailment: Health Care." *Time*, Nov. 11, 1991.

Lessenberry, Jack. "Death Becomes Him." *Vanity Fair*, July 1993. Reprinted on www.pbs.org/wgbh/pages/frontline/kevorkian/aboutk/vanityfair.htm.

Marchione, Marilyn. "Conquering the Killers." Associated Press, April 11, 2005.

Matalin, Mary, and James Carville. *All's Fair: Love, War and Running for President*. New York: Random House, 1994.

McMurray, Colleen. "Number of Teen Smokers Holding Steady." Gallup Poll News Service, May 18, 2004.

Mooney, Elizabeth C. "The White Plague." *American Heritage* 30, no. 2 (February–March 1979).

Porter, Roy. *The Greatest Benefit to Mankind: A Medical History of Humanity*. New York: W. W. Norton, 1997.

Prichard, Oliver, Sandy Bauers, and Larry Fish. "A 'Calm, Peaceful' End Amid a Bitter Dispute." *Philadelphia Inquirer*, April 1, 2005.

"Public Sees Smoking Linked to Lung Cancer, Poll Reveals." Public Opinion News Service, July 21, 1957.

Quadagno, Jill. "Why the United States Has No National Health Insurance." *Journal of Health and Social Behavior* 45 (2004).

Schwartz, John. "New Openness in Deciding When and How to Die." *New York Times*, March 21, 2005.

Stout, Hillary. "Many Don't Realize It's Clinton's Plan They Like." *Wall Street Journal*, March 10, 1994.

"U.S. Public Divides About Evenly on Cigarette-Heart Disease Link." Public Opinion News Service, July 24, 1957.

Vitez, Michael. "9 to 5 till . . . 95?" *Philadelphia Inquirer*, May 29, 2005.

REPORTS

U.S. Centers for Disease Control and Prevention. *Morbidity and Mortality Weekly Report* 50, no. 21 (June 1, 2001): 433–34.

INTERNET SOURCES

"Electric Heart," transcript from *NOVA* broadcast, Dec. 21, 1999.
http://www.pbs.org/wgbh/nova/transcripts/2617eheart.html

"A Few of Our Losses."
http://www.tobacco.org/resources/misc/losses.html

Gallup Poll, June 29–July 4, 1950.
http://brain.gallup.com/documents

"Influenza 1918."
http://www.pbs.org/wgbh/amex/influenza/peopleevents/pandeAMEX
90.html

"Inside the Tobacco Deal." *Frontline*, May 1998.
http://www.pbs.org/wgbh/pages/frontline/shows/settlement/
interviews/

"The Medical Treatment of Disease."
http://www.umanitoba.ca/faculties/medicine/history/notes/
treatment/

"Patient Gets First Totally Implanted Artificial Heart." CNN.com
Health
http://archives.cnn.com/2001/HEALTH/conditions/07/03/artificial.
heart/

"Pioneering Artificial Heart Patient Dies." Associated Press, Nov. 30,
2001
http://www.usatoday.com/news/nation/2001/11/30/heart.htm.

"Robert Koch and Tuberculosis."
http://nobelprize.org/medicine/educational/tuberculosis/
readmore.html

"Whatever Happened to Polio?" Smithsonian National Museum of
American History
http://americanhistory.si.edu/polio/americanepi/families.htm

ALZHEIMER'S ASSOCIATION
225 N. Michigan Ave., Floor 17
Chicago, IL 60601-7633
(800) 272-3900
Website: www.alz.org

The Alzheimer's Association is one of America's largest advocacy groups for sufferers of Alzheimer's disease and for their caregivers.

AMERICAN MEDICAL ASSOCIATION
515 N. State St.
Chicago, IL 60610
(800) 621-8335
Website: www.ama-assn.org

The national organization representing American physicians takes positions on a number of public health issues, including cigarette smoking, the cost of health care, the education of doctors, underage drinking, and a patients' bill of rights.

CAMPAIGN FOR TOBACCO-FREE KIDS
1400 Eye St., Suite 1200
Washington, DC 20005
(202) 296-5469
Website: http://tobaccofreekids.org

The organization has prepared many studies on tobacco use by young people that can be accessed at its website. It has identified and described a number of federal and state initiatives that are aimed at reducing the availability of cigarettes to teenagers.

COMPASSION IN DYING FEDERATION
6312 SW Capitol Highway, Suite 415
Portland, OR 97239
(503) 221-9556
Website: www.compassionindying.org

The organization counsels people who are facing end-of-life choices due to medical conditions; the group's website provides an overview of the rights guaranteed to terminally ill patients.

NATIONAL COALITION ON HEALTH CARE

1200 G St., NW, Suite 750
Washington, DC 20005
(202) 638-7151
Website: www.nchc.org

This nonprofit and bipartisan organization studies the rising cost of health care and recommends ways that costs can be reined in; statistics and reports on the impact of health care costs on Americans can be downloaded at the organization's website.

POST-POLIO HEALTH INTERNATIONAL

4207 Lindell Blvd., No. 110
St. Louis, MO 63108-2915
(314) 534-0475
Website: www.post-polio.org

As many as 180,000 Americans who survived polio may still display symptoms of the disease; the organization serves as an advocacy and support group for them.

U.S. CENTERS FOR DISEASE CONTROL AND PREVENTION

Office of Communication
Building 16, D-42
1600 Clifton Rd., NE
Atlanta, GA 30333
(800) 311-3435
Website: www.cdc.gov

Numerous reports and studies on treatments, diseases, and other health issues are available on the website maintained by the federal government's chief public health agency.

Numbers in **bold italics** refer to captions.

For almost three-quarters of a century, the GALLUP POLL has measured the attitudes and opinions of the American public about the major events and the most important political, social, and economic issues of the day. Founded in 1935 by Dr. George Gallup, the Gallup Poll was the world's first public opinion poll based on scientific sampling procedures. For most of its history, the Gallup Poll was sponsored by the nation's largest newspapers, which published two to four of Gallup's public opinion reports each week. Poll findings, which covered virtually every major news event and important issue facing the nation and the world, were reported in a variety of media. More recently, the poll has been conducted in partnership with CNN and USA Today. All of Gallup's findings, including many opinion trends dating back to the 1930s and 1940s, are accessible at www.gallup.com.

ALEC M. GALLUP is chairman of The Gallup Poll in the United States, and Chairman of The Gallup Organization Ltd. in Great Britain. He also serves as a director of The Gallup Organisation, Europe; Gallup China; and Gallup Hungary. He has been employed by Gallup since 1959 and has directed or played key roles in many of the company's most ambitious and innovative projects, including Gallup's 2002 "Survey of Nine Islamic Nations"; the "Global Cities Project"; the "Global Survey on Attitudes Towards AIDS"; the 25-nation "Health of The Planet Survey"; and the ongoing "Survey of Consumer Attitudes and Lifestyles in China." Mr. Gallup also oversees several annual "social audits," including "Black and White Relations in the United States," an investigation of attitudes and perceptions concerning the state of race relations, and "Survey of the Public's Attitudes Toward the Public Schools," which tracks attitudes on educational issues.

Mr. Gallup's educational background includes undergraduate work at Princeton University and the University of Iowa. He undertook graduate work in communications and journalism at Stanford University, and studied marketing and advertising research at New York University. His publications include *The Great American Success Story* (with George Gallup, Jr.; Dow Jones-Irwin, 1986), *Presidential Approval: A Source Book* (with George Edwards; Johns Hopkins University Press, 1990), *The Gallup Poll Cumulative Index: Public Opinion* 1935–1997 (Scholarly Resources, 1999), and *British Political Opinion 1937–2000: The Gallup Polls* (with Anthony King and Robert Wybrow; Politicos Publishing, 2001).

HAL MARCOVITZ has written more than 70 books for young readers. His other titles in the GALLUP MAJOR TRENDS & EVENTS series include *Technology, Race Relations, Drug and Alcohol Abuse*, and *Abortion*. He lives in Chalfont, Pennsylvania, with his wife Gail and daughters Ashley and Michelle. In addition to writing nonfiction, he enjoys writing fiction and is the author of the satirical novel *Painting the White House*.